Osteoporosis:
The Silent Stalker

The Woman's Illustrated Health Care Guide to Preventing and Reversing Osteoporosis

by

Dr. Timothy J. Gray

Illustrated by Kathy Kaplan, R.N.

BookPartners, Inc.
Wilsonville, Oregon

Ogen is a registered trademark of Abbott Corp., N. Chicago, IL
Premarin is a registered trademark of Wyeth-Ayerst Corp., Philadelphia, PA
Estrace is a registered trademark of Mead-Johnson Corp., Princeton, NJ
Estraderm is a registered trademark of Ciba Corp., Woodbridge, NJ
Amen is a registered trademark of Carnrick Corp., Cedar Knolls, NJ
Provera is a registered trademark of Upjohn Corp., Kalamazoo, MI
Cycrin is a registered trademark of Wyeth-Ayerst Corp., Philadelphia, PA
Nautilus is a registered trademark of Nautilus Corp., Independence, VA
Dirk Pitt is a character in the novel *Sahara* written by Clive Cussler.

BookPartners, Inc.
P.O. Box 922
Wilsonville, Oregon 97070

Dedication

This book is dedicated to my mother, Kathleen Gray, for her encouragement, her support and her unending efforts to give us every possible opportunity for education and for the love of learning she instilled into our young minds.

To Peter whose footsteps over the years have grown so large that I couldn't fill them. With his help I was able to continue school when I wasn't sure where the next dollar was coming from.

To Mary Beth whose values transcend the physical and who balances our lives with higher values.

To John who is spending his life making life better for others. His understanding of situations and people is uncanny and his ideas always seem to produce marvelous results.

To Kevin whose world travels open up our minds to other cultures and ideas for living.

To Kathy who has the ability to turn complicated concepts into visual images through her use of several art forms.

To Charles who never gives up even against insurmountable odds. His courage encourages us.

To Suzanne whose zest for life and adventures keeps us all wondering: what next?

Acknowledgements

I wish to personally thank David Rianda from the Northwest Osteopathic Foundation who started the entire project on osteoporosis. A special thanks to Carla Weiting R.N., who coordinated the television program on osteoporosis and whose easy, organized manner allowed the material to flow smoothly.

A special thank you to my family; Kathy, T.J., Tom and Laura who accepted the piles of books and articles that filled our home and for Laura posing for the pictures in the book.

Thanks to Faye Fresh R.N., Nancy Dober L.P.N., Laura Hanchett R.N., Pam Wild R.N., Ms. Heather Bolen,for giving their time to creating visual images of medical concepts, Dr. Greg Damery for his technical assistance, and Dee Michaud for her assistance in the clinic.

Thanks for the cooperation of Jenine Vrtiska, the project coordinator, and Rayberta Jenkins, Carmen Reed and Tina Dean who kept our medical facility functioning during the growing phase of the book's birth. Karen Kirwan R.N., F.N.P.-C. has enthusiastically developed the position of women's health specialist during the diagnosis and treatment phases of osteoporosis evaluation. Shanna Midland helped with research as did Natalie Norcross, the Tuality Hospital Medical Librarian. Thanks to Jim Surface P.T., for helping to develop exercise protocols for the different stages of osteoporosis. Thanks to Ursula and Thorn Bacon for their untiring efforts to make the manuscript read smoothly and for the cover design, and to Sheryl Mehary for her skills in word processing. And finally, I express my gratitude to Sheryn Hara who continues to spread the book information to reader groups across the country and across international boundaries.

Leonardo da Vinci's "A Cannon of Proportions"

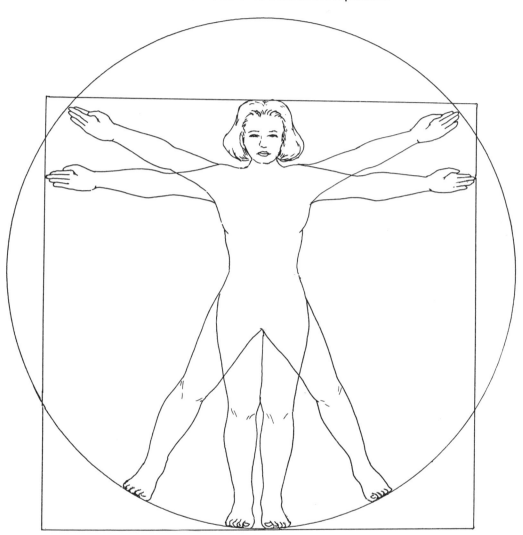

In the early 1600s Leonardo da Vinci diagnosed osteoporosis by comparing the proportions of women. Normally the height of any individual equals the span from fingertip to fingertip. Da Vinci concluded that when a woman's height was less than her width of arm span, then she was suffering from compression fractures and as a consequence her body height shortened.

Table Of Contents

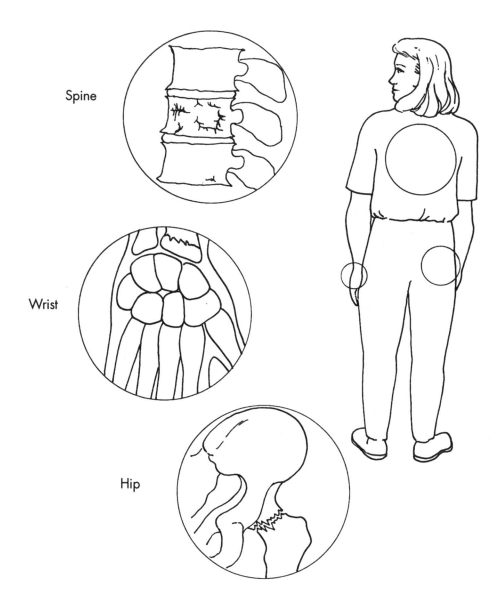

Spine

Wrist

Hip

Illustration 1 – Areas affected by osteoporosis

Introduction

Osteoporosis. It's called the silent stalker of women. One out of four women have it, yet most are unaware of it. It's a robber of health that begins in the teens, reaches crisis proportions after menopause and causes havoc with women's lives during the Golden Years.

For many women, the golden years mean gold fillings and gold charge cards for medical expenses. But financial security cannot prevent women from losing their independence and often their lives to osteoporosis — a disease that is absolutely preventable.

That's the message of this book. Osteoporosis is preventable. You don't have to be a victim if you follow some straightforward medical advice.

Pap smears have cut the incidence of cancer of the cervix. Mammography has dramatically increased survival from breast cancer because of early detection and early treatment when it is most effective. Women have diets to lower fat and cholesterol to save their hearts.

Yet, osteoporosis is a bigger problem than all the feminine cancers and heart diseases put together! Over one million women will suffer fractures of the spine, the hips or other bones this year from osteoporosis. Half of those will be spine fractures. One fourth of them will be hip fractures. Only ten percent of the women with hip fractures will return to a normal life. Twenty percent will die the first year of complications and many of the others will end up in a nursing home. Osteoporosis dissolves bones and robs women of vitality at a time in life when they should be enjoying the greatest amount of freedom.

Our bones are like a savings account. We put calcium into them over the years and when we need the calcium, it will be there for us. Trying to play the catch up game with calcium is difficult. It's like trying to retire on savings put away between 55 and 65. It's almost impossible to put away enough cash in ten years to live comfortably. The same is true of calcium. Women with osteoporosis feel tired. The common complaint doctors hear is: "I'm sick and tired of being sick and tired." The bones are overworked for the strength they have; the muscles are weak. Most women with symptoms of osteoporosis have difficulty lifting ten pounds!

This book is a common-sense approach to one of the great problems of our time. The first chapter is written by a woman who was my patient. She suffered from osteoporosis and recovered, following instruction I gave her. She told me that she was so shaken by her close encounter with health disaster that she wanted to warn other women about the hazards of neglecting to protect themselves against osteoporosis. When she learned that I was writing a book for women on osteoporosis, she suggested that her letter to me entitled: *A Message To All My Sisters* would make a good beginning.

I agree with her. It is a warning to women, and it is a confirmation that good health care practices women anywhere can follow will prevent the silent stalker from touching their lives.

... 1 ...

A Message To All My Sisters

Dear Sisters:

I want to spare you the pain I'm going through. It started in my teens when I was reading fashion magazines. The models with their long, slender legs, tiny waists and curving bodies caught my eye. I wanted to be like them. Their life style was appealing. Pictures of them posing in front of the Eiffel Tower or strolling the isolated beaches under palm trees caught my heart. I decided to look like they did.

I had no idea how to become a model. The few extra pounds I had on my hips seemed resistant to exercise so I began dieting and fasting. No dairy products for me; too much fat. I didn't even stop to think that they were a prime source of calcium. I just didn't eat them.

At 5' 4" inches, I weighed 100 pounds. Looking in the mirror I saw what nobody else could see. I saw fat. My parents and family physician told me that I was ten pounds underweight but I didn't believe them. I kept dieting constantly to keep the extra pounds off. I never became a model because I always felt fat.

When I was pregnant with my daughter, I gained only 10 pounds. The doctor said I needed to add more weight. I didn't. At birth Sarah weighed 9 pounds. I tried to take calcium supplements during pregnancy, but I became constipated so I discontinued them.

Nursing my daughter and watching her grow was so exciting for me. I didn't take the calcium then either. I was bewitched when Sarah's little hands held my finger and she'd fall asleep in my arms. Life was beautiful.

As she grew, we enjoyed Bluebirds and Campfire Girls together. Her front teeth fell out, then new ones came in crookedly, only to be straightened with braces. I wanted her to have everything I could give her.

I was always present for her soccer and basketball games in the fall and winter and for softball games in the spring. At her high school graduation I was so proud of her. She stood tall and straight with her flowing gown and mortar board cap. Then she was gone …

An emptiness filled the house and my spirit. What would I do without her? It took a long time to get used to the empty chair and the stuffed animals that stayed on her bed instead of cluttering the house.

When Sarah graduated from high school I began having some symptoms. My gums hurt and were soft and sore — the first indication of periodontal disease. The dentist became the other man in my life. Flossing and mixing pastes, massaging and rubbing my gums was my new hobby. I was trying to keep my teeth. I didn't know at the time that periodontal or gum disease is an early sign of osteoporosis for many women. It is often called osteoporosis of the mouth.

I didn't know what osteoporosis was. Then I began to find out about the silent stalker. Osteoporosis is an upset body chemistry with more bone loss that bone production. Osteo means bone. Porosis means porous. Porous, weakened, brittle bones are the result.

I thought that gum disease just happened. Didn't everybody have gum problems and bone and back pain at my age? Weren't leg and foot cramping normal for a forty-two-year- old? Why was I so tired all the time? Why did Sarah look taller all the time?

One morning I was making coffee and looked at the back of my hand and saw my mother's skin on my hand. I was becoming my mother. The thin, shiny skin on the back of my hand couldn't be my skin; there had to be a mistake. Something was wrong. That thin, shiny skin was my mother's skin and she had osteoporosis.

"Was my shiny skin related to my hysterectomy seven years ago when I was 35?" I asked myself.

I went to see Dr. Gray, a big affable man who is our family doctor. I told him about my symptoms and he scolded me gently for stopping my estrogen after my hysterectomy and for avoiding calcium. I told him that the estrogen didn't seem to do anything except diminish the hot flashes a little, so I stopped taking it when the first bottle was empty.

He said. "It sounds like you are developing osteoporosis." Your bones are getting soft.

I asked. "How can that be?"

Dr. Gray gave me a pamphlet about osteoporosis. Page two showed the risk factors and I couldn't help but apply them to myself. At risk were females of an older age (I wasn't THAT old!), who experienced early menopause as a result of hysterectomy. White race was another determinant (I was white). Low calcium intake was a factor (I gulped). Physical inactivity was cited. (What did they mean physical inactivity? I had a full-time job and took care of our home.) Low body weight was an important sign. (I thought being thin was good—that fat was the enemy.) A family history of osteoporosis was an early warning to heed. (My mother is bent forward when she walks.) And smoking (I don't smoke!)was a determinant, as was excess alcohol consumption (I rarely drink).

I was angry. "Why me?" I asked. "I'm a good person who does the right things in life."

Dr. Gray explained that osteoporosis isn't a moral issue, but is a biochemical problem in which bone mass is lost. "Your job," he said, "is to start taking steps to reverse the process."   "How can I do that?" I asked.

He pointed out that I was in the early stages of osteoporosis and there was time to treat the problem. He recommended weight-bearing activities like jogging, walking, tennis, bicycling, dancing, cross-country skiing, weight training and aerobics.

He spoke eloquently about the value of exercise. He said that bone mass and strength are related to the muscle mass and that I could control my muscle mass and strength with exercise. He said, "To keep your bones hard, you must keep your muscles hard."

Then, he gave me the Bicep Test. He asked me to make a muscle in my arm. "Now squeeze it," he said. I did squeeze it between my thumb and index finger and made a big dent in the skin.

"That's not good." Doctor Gray said, observing the soft indentation. "Your

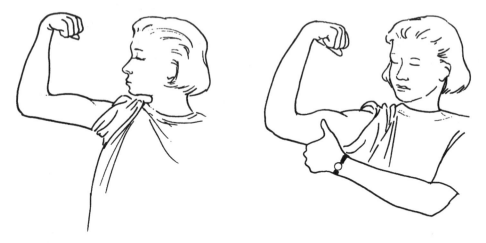

Illustration 2 – Bicep Test.

bicep muscle gives you an idea about your general muscle strength. The muscle should be firm." While he was speaking, I noticed for the first time some skin hanging down below my upper arm, just like my mother had. I couldn't believe it.

"Get out and start exercising." Dr. Gray said. "Use it or lose it, as the old adage goes. Follow the SAFE program of exercise. SAFE stands for strength, aerobics, flexibility and endurance."

I wasn't sure exactly how to start the SAFE program, so he referred me to the local health facility, *Vitality and Fitness*. He gave me a written exercise prescription that I stuck on my refrigerator door.

The trainers were excellent. They showed me which machines to use to strengthen my muscles overall while protecting my back. I joined an aerobics class and stretched every day. Dr. Gray said that weight bearing exercises were the best exercises to promote bone stress and bone hardening. The exercise gym had treadmills, bikes and step machines. I tried them all and loved the variety. I learned how to use them safely.

During this time as I was beginning to feel renewed, my mother fell and fractured her wrist. It was a common fracture that happens frequently with persons who are suffering from osteoporosis, her doctor told her. The wrist fracture was a mild problem compared to the vertebral or spinal fractures that happened to her. Also,

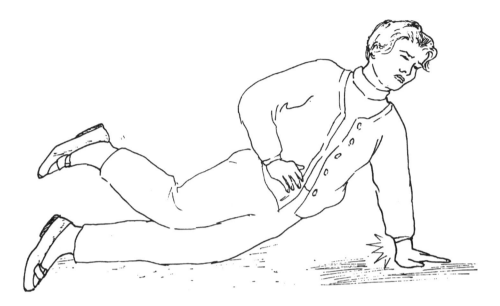

Illustration 3 – Falling On Wrist.

Mom had lost several inches of height, typical of women who become bent with the disease. As a rule, I learned, women lose 1-1/2 inches of height for each decade of life beginning at menopause around age 50 or sooner if you've had a hysterectomy and aren't making or taking estrogen.

I was astonished to discover that osteoporosis is responsible for 90 percent of all fractures in women who are over the age of 55. Osteoporosis causes more problems and deaths than all of the heart diseases and feminine cancers combined. I couldn't believe that it hadn't been brought to the attention of women sooner.

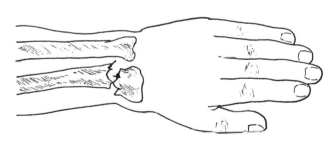

Illustration 4 – Broken Wrist.

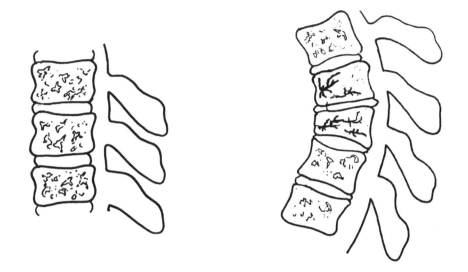

Illustration 5 – Healthy Vertebrae and Anterior Compression Fractures.

My mother recovered from her wrist fracture. I invited her to come with me to the exercise gym but she said her doctor wanted her to attend a special physical therapy program first to learn how to exercise without hurting her brittle bones. She was started on a gentle stretching program using therabands, rubberized sport bands of different colors for increasing resistance. Slowly she improved to the point that she and I could have workouts together. Her workout, of course, was less intense.

I wanted to learn more about osteoporosis, the robber of health, so I went to the public library. I took out all the books I could find. I researched magazine articles and I came across a questionnaire in a women's magazine. I wished I had seen it 20 years ago. It asked these questions of readers:

One In Four Women Get Osteoporosis — Will You?

Take this quick test to see.   Check yes or no

1. Are you caucasian or asian?   _____ _____
2. Do you smoke or live with a smoker?   _____ _____
3. Do you drink alcohol daily?   _____ _____
4. Do you drink more than 2 cups of coffee daily?   _____ _____
5. Do you have relatives with osteoporosis?   _____ _____
6. Are you underweight for your height?.   _____ _____
    See the weight table on page 14.
7. Have you stopped having periods for reasons other than
    pregnancy or nursing?   _____ _____
8. Have you taken cortisone medications for more than a few
    months?   _____ _____
9. Do you perform less than one hour of weight bearing
    (walking, aerobics or weight lifting) exercises per week?   _____ _____
10. Are you allergic or intolerant of dairy products?   _____ _____

SCORING.   1-3 yes answers = average risk of osteoporosis
                4-6 yes answers = above average risk
                7-10 yes answers = severe potential problems

I discovered that women who scored with four or more yes answers needed to restructure their approach to exercise, and diet and to investigate, as I did, an altered life-style. Failure to do so would put them in a high risk of osteoporosis category.

Estrogen, I learned from my reading is the key element in preventing and treating osteoporosis. Over one million fractures are caused each year in women whose bones have been weakened by osteoporosis. Of the quarter million women who fracture a hip each year, only ten percent will ever return to normal activity. I was aghast! These statistics were frightening! One half a million vertebral fractures and one third million fractures of ribs, pelvis and other bones happened to women who become needless victims of the silent stalker.

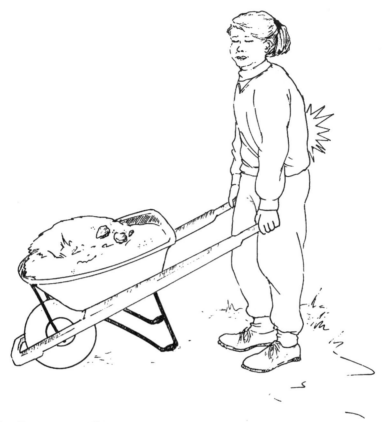

Illustration 6 – Compression Fracture.

The Incredible Shrinking Woman

I discovered the value of estrogen when I heard the story of Mary from Dr. Gray. Mary was 60, working in her yard loading debris into the wheelbarrow. Once full, she lifted the wheelbarrow as she had done thousands of times when she heard a loud snap in her back. She felt as if she had been stabbed with a kitchen knife. Excruciating pain bowled her over and muscle spasms came and went for weeks. She took narcotic pain medications to control the pain of the compression fracture. Two months later she crushed another vertebra when she stepped off a high curb. Recovery for Mary was slower the second time.

As a result of her fractures, Mary's body height dropped several inches. She

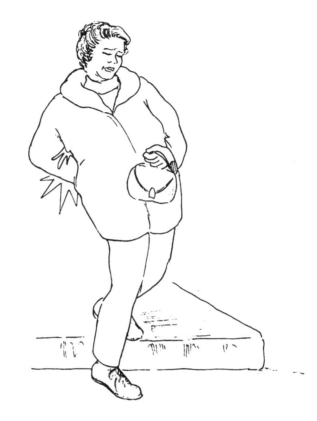

Illustration 7 – Another Compression Fracture.

shrank. Her upper back was stooped forward and her rib cage almost touched her pelvis. Mary withdrew from her friends and family. Her self-esteem plummeted and she became depressed. She avoided her friends and refused dinner invitations from friends at public restaurants. So stooped was Mary that she felt gnome-like with her face hovering above her plate. Her abdomen protruded excessively from the bent-forward position. When she was able to find clothes that fit her around the middle, they would be too large for the rest of her body. Mary despaired. She had always loved dressing nicely but now was unable to shop in normal clothing stores and had to make baggy shifts that would hang loosely like a sheet draped over a chair in an abandoned house.

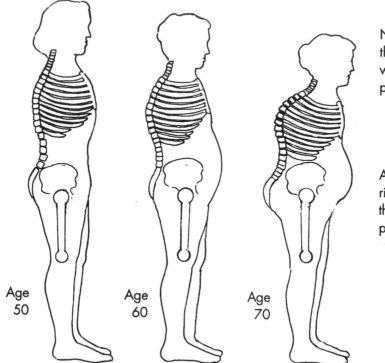

Notice at age 60, as the chest bends forward the abdomen protrudes.

At Age 70, now the ribs touch on pelvis – the abdomen always protrudes.

Age 50   Age 60   Age 70

Illustration 8 – Progressive Spinal Deformity in Osteoporosis.

Psychological counseling and antidepressants were prescribed for Mary. They helped her to accept her condition and deal with it. Did Mary have any early-warning signs of her coming disfiguration? No, she didn't, but she did have symptoms of estrogen deficiency that occur at the menopause. She remembered hot flashes and sweats, vaginal dryness, urinary tract infections, depression, mood swings and breast shrinkage, but unfortunately she accepted these changes as part of the aging process. I learned that women don't have to accept these changes. They can be effectively prevented and treated.

In a family with a history of osteoporosis, estrogen deficiency is a warning sign that the problem is present. What can we do? My library research and my dozens of questions to Doctor Gray on osteoporosis have helped me to develop ten commandments:

The 10 Commandments To Prevent Osteoporosis

1. Eat plenty of calcium-rich foods.
2. Limit alcohol, caffeine and soda pop.
3. Avoid fasting diets.
4. Exercise at least four times a week.
5. Take estrogen post-menopause if you are high risk.
6. Avoid excess thyroid medication, it softens the bones.
7. Avoid smoke either first or second hand.
8. Listen to your doctor regarding treatment options.
9. Spend less time in your easy chair.
10. Perform weight bearing activities.

What about the women who already have osteoporosis? Is there hope for them? Yes, there is hope for women whose bones are breaking and whose life styles have been drastically altered. See a physician to get an estimate of your condition. Depending on how far the disease has progressed, improvement in your health can be achieved. Remember my mother?

Request bone density measurements from your doctor to determine how hard your bones are. The test needs to be repeated from time to time to monitor your response to exercise and therapy.

I have written this letter to all my sisters to encourage you to take action now in your life. There is nothing more sorrowful than a woman who has aged prematurely, who has grown old, and looks old and bowed when it absolutely isn't necessary.

Somehow women are still trapped in the old fashioned idea that aging means loss of their vitality, their sexual powers, their softness, their femininity. That's non-sense! It's an old wive's tale arising out of ignorance and misinformation. Preserve your womanhood and your beauty by following the simple steps of prevention.

I want you to avoid the pain I'm going through. I've stopped my bones from softening with my new life style of exercise and sensible eating. I get my calcium and I take estrogen since I've already lost 21 percent of my bone mass as measured on a DEXA scan.

Stay fit, eat wisely and give your body one hour of exercise daily. You have plenty of time to firm up your bones. Remember to check your bicep muscle to see how you are doing.

Are You Underweight for Your Height?

Use the simple formula doctors use to determine your ideal weight.

Small Frame		Medium Frame		Large Frame	
Height	Weight	Height	Weight	Height	Weight
4' 10"	90#	4' 10"	100#	4' 10"	110#
4' 11"	95#	4" 11"	105#	4' 11"	115#
5' 0"	100#	5' 0"	110#	5' 0"	120#
5' 1"	105#	5' 1"	115#	5' 1"	125#
5' 2"	110#	5' 2"	120#	5' 2"	130#
5" 3"	115#	5' 3"	125#	5' 3"	135#
5' 4"	120#	5' 4"	130#	5' 4"	140#
5' 5"	125#	5' 5"	135#	5' 5"	145#
5' 6"	130#	5' 6"	140#	5' 6"	150#
5' 7"	135#	5' 7"	145#	5' 7"	155#
5' 8"	140#	5' 8"	150#	5' 8"	160#
5' 9"	145#	5' 9"	155#	5' 9"	165#
5' 10"	150#	5' 10"	160#	5' 10"	170#
5' 11"	155#	5' 11"	165#	5' 11'	175#
6" 0"	160#	6' 0"	170#	6' 0"	180#
6' 1"	165#	6' 1"	175#	6' 1"	185#
6' 2"	170#	6' 2"	180#	6' 2"	190#

The formula used for these measurements is based on a five foot tall woman with a thin body build who should weigh 100 pounds. For each extra inch add 5 pounds. A medium weight woman should weigh 110 pounds for 5 feet of height and add 5 pounds for each extra inch. A large frame woman should weigh 120 pounds for five feet in height and add 5 pounds for each additional inch in height.

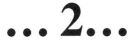

Diagnostic Tests

We know much more about osteoporosis today than when I studied the disease in medical school. Quite recent groundbreaking research by Dr. John Eisman of the Garvan Institute of Medical Research in Sydney, Australia has given us new information that indicates that genes in the body influence a form of Vitamin D which plays a crucial role in bone formation. In a report to Nature Magazine, the researchers, led by Dr. Eisman, said they discovered two versions of a specific gene which are associated with the bone density a person inherits. One type, which they labeled "b" is linked to stronger skeletons, and one, labeled "B" is associated with weaker ones.

The importance of this discovery when it is verified by more research is to make it easier for physicians to discover earlier if a patient has a sturdy or weak bone profile. Such knowledge will act as a warning to the "B" type individual that she needs to be more cautious about the risk factors in her physical makeup that may lead her to osteoporosis if they are ignored.

It will be nice when the day comes that a woman can be tested for her risk of osteoporosis. In Dr. Eisman's words, "I envision a woman going in for a blood test which will become as routine as a cholesterol check to assess her bone density and risk for osteoporosis."

What would such a test actually tell you? It would inform you of the genetic information you received from your parents specifically related to osteoporosis.

Yes, the individual risk of osteoporosis depends absolutely on heredity. Each of your parents contribute a copy of the receptor gene which controls a form of Vitamin D. This important vitamin apparently influences calcium absorption and the renewal of bone. If each of your parents give you two little b's, the type of genetic endowment that favors strong bones, you're in great shape. But if you're unlucky enough to have parents who supply you with two big B's, then you've inherited the double danger of the low-bone-density form of the gene. You're definitely at risk of having osteoporosis by the time you reach 65.

While it's always informative to know about new medical advances, the Australian research and its enthusiastic reception by the medical community in America stresses the significance physicians attach to osteoporosis as a health threat. And while we don't have the diagnostic blood test for osteoporosis yet, the emphasis on osteoporosis research reminds us of the necessity to warn women to avail themselves of existing testing procedures.

You'll learn about these tests in this chapter. The important thing for women to remember in view of the fact that one in four females in America will develop osteoporosis, is that the disease offers no early symptoms. That puts the responsibility for discovery upon you. If you are between the ages of 35and 55, that's the age bracket when you want to be medically evaluated.

But before we look at the tests available for the disease, let's take a look at the three stages of osteoporosis and how women are affected. As we examine the stages of the disease's development, try to place yourself in the appropriate category, then design a program based on the information in this book and advice from your physician to reverse the process.

Stage I – Before Symptoms
Stage One is symptomless. Clarice was classified in this category, but what did we know about her? She was 36 years old, with fair skin, was 5'5" tall and weighed 117 pounds. She had epilepsy and took Dilantin medication to prevent seizures. Clarice smoked one pack of cigarettes per day, drank five or six soft drinks in a 24 hour period and had an occasional glass of wine. She took no calcium supplements but she did eat low-fat dairy products. In the past she took birth control pills. Clarice was an

adopted child and was unaware of her family history. She made no effort to exercise regularly.

Because of the risk factors she exhibited, her anti-convulsant medication, her smoking habit, increased intake of caffeine in soft drinks, thin body build, and minimal exercise, I knew she was a candidate for osteoporosis.

Testing showed Clarice had a bone mineral content normal for her age. Despite the risk factors she demonstrated, Clarice reached bone maturity with a normal amount of bone mass, probably aided by the estrogen replacement chemicals in the birth control pills she took.

Because of her need for long-term treatment with anti- convulsants, Clarice was at increased risk for bone loss. She was advised to join a women's health club and use Nautilus equipment and to participate in low-impact aerobics. These activities are part of the treatment for patients without symptoms or fractures, but who may be contributing to osteoporosis risk as a result of medication, diet or hereditary factors. See Chapter Six on gym exercise.

Nancy was 38 years old, had a thin body build and smoked two packs of cigarettes per day. She had a history of an ulcer and had been taking aluminum-containing antacids for years. She did not exercise. Two of her relatives had fractures of the spine from osteoporosis.

Testing showed a bone mineral content below average for her age suggesting that Nancy was a candidate for spontaneous fractures. She was counseled to change the risk factors that she could control. She was referred to a smoking cessation clinic, started on a walking program and given antacids without aluminum to control her ulcer symptoms. She was advised to use TUMS since they contain calcium and would help treat her bones while she was treating her ulcer.

Another strong suspect for osteoporosis was Danette, 40 years old, 5'4" who weighed 125 pounds. The mother of two, she had been on thyroid medication for years. Her 66-year-old mother exhibited classic osteoporosis bone changes. She had suffered compression fractures of the spine and had developed a stooped back and posture. Danette drank three or four glasses of wine daily; she walked, jogged and participated in aerobics three times weekly. Because of her family history, she was tested carefully and it was revealed that her bone density to be slightly below average.

Danette's family history, her thyroid medication and her alcohol intake put her at risk for a fracture. Placed on 1500 mg of calcium daily and advised to decrease her alcohol intake, Danette was also informed that she should consider estrogen therapy when her menopause occurred particularly if her bone density was decreasing at that time.

Stage II – Symptoms Begin

Stage two of osteoporosis signifies that a woman may have noticed bodily changes like gum disease, thin skin on the back of her hands, bone pain, fatigue or hot flashes. These changes should be your diagnostic early warning signs. They tell you that your body is beginning to succumb to loss of bone strength. Take steps to stop the loss of bone now.

Pam is a woman with a family history of osteoporosis. Trim, 58, 5'2" in height, weighing 112 pounds with a history of a hysterectomy, Pam exercised occasionally with Nautilus machines, the treadmill and the step machine. Her mother walked with a cane after a hip fracture. Pam was afraid that she would develop fractures since she noticed thin skin on the back of her hands. Leg and foot cramps at night worried her. Sometimes cramps like hers are a sign of excess calcium movement out of the bone into the bloodstream and out the kidneys. She hadn't taken estrogen but had been taking 1500 mg of calcium daily since menopause from surgery.

Pam knew that if 1500 mg of calcium was good for her, 5000 mg of calcium was not. Vitamins and minerals taken in excess may be toxic to the system. She was wise in monitoring her dosage. Excess calcium can cause kidney stones, severe constipation or abnormal heart rhythms. Read Chapter Three on calcium to learn how to use calcium appropriately.

Her family history of osteoporosis made Pam anxious and as a result she was tested thoroughly with a QCT scan. That was the only test available in her community. The computer printout showed clearly that for her age her bone condition was poor.

Discouraged, she decided her lifestyle wasn't healthy enough. Most bone loss normally occurs by about age 60 or 65, so Pam was worried that at 58, she was still not past the most critical stage of bone loss.

She was encouraged to exercise on a daily basis with weight-bearing activities. See Chapter Six. An estrogen/progesterone combination was prescribed for her until age 65 and she was advised to keep her Vitamin D intake at 400 units daily.

Another Stage Two woman was Judy, a 67-year-old Asian woman, short and slim with two grown children and an aunt with a wrist fracture from osteoporosis. Judy

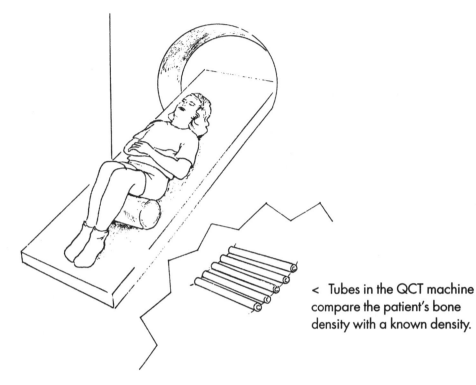

< Tubes in the QCT machine compare the patient's bone density with a known density.

Illustration 9 – Quantitative Computed Tomography (QCT).

underwent menopause at 47 due to a hysterectomy. She took estrogen for a decade following her menopause but hadn't taken any for the immediate past 10 years. Judy walked two miles per week and worked in a small shop making floral arrangements. She did not smoke or drink but felt chronically tired and had bone pain in the back and legs.

It was discovered that Judy's bone mineral content was well below normal for her age and a 24-hour urine calcium test indicated that she was losing more calcium than she was taking in. The calcium was slowly being drained from her bones.

We encouraged Judy to exercise by walking at lunch daily. Since she was a home-body we recommended the home exercise program. See Chapter Seven. Judy's doctor prescribed a combination of estrogen and testosterone which has been shown to increase bone mass after menopause. The low dose testosterone gave her renewed vigor and hope that she could avoid the complications of back and hip fractures.

Stage III - The Fractures

Once fractures occur, immediate therapy is indicated! This final stage sets the background for tremendous pain, medical expenses and personal frustration. Bicycles and hiking shoes are replaced with walkers and braces while evenings with friends are replaced with lonely, agonizing hours. Work around the house or yard which normally takes four hours, requires 12 hours if you can do it at all. Driving a car becomes a nightmare as you try to see over the steering wheel with your slumped back. Don't give up when problems start, there is hope.

Let's examine two women, Carrie and Beth, both in stage three.

Carrie was 67, Hispanic, and had a hysterectomy in her late forties. She had no hormonal therapy and exhibited constant back pain from crushed vertebral fractures. See page 20. She was being treated with low dose testosterone to prevent losing more than the five inches of height that had already shortened her stature. Carrie had smoked two packs a day for forty years.

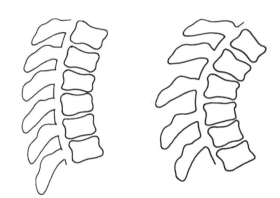

Illustration 10 – Vertebrae; Normal and After Compression Fractures.

With bone density tests indicating deterioration in her body, Carrie had no desire to become an invalid. She was told that spinal fracture usually preceded hip fractures by a few years and she was at high risk.

She agreed to being treated with Didronel and calcium. Didronel hardens the bones more than estrogen and is given in two month cycles alternating with calcium. In addition,

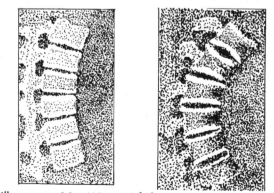

Illustration 11 – X-Rays Of The Same Vertebrae as Above.

— 20 —

Carrie started on a walking program daily and started rehabilitation on a supervised program. See pages 21 to 27. She started using prescription nicotine patches to help her stop smoking. She said she would rather pay for medication and earn another chance at life through exercise than pay the money to a nursing home as her body dwindled.

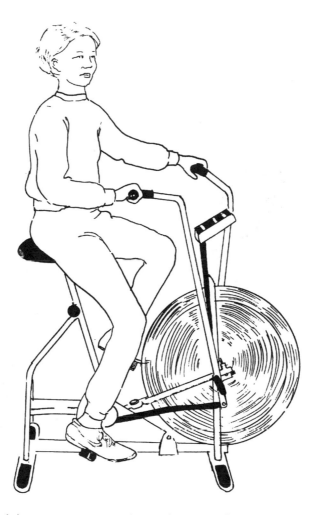

Illustration 12 – Rehabilitation, Stationary Bike – Schwinn Airdyne.

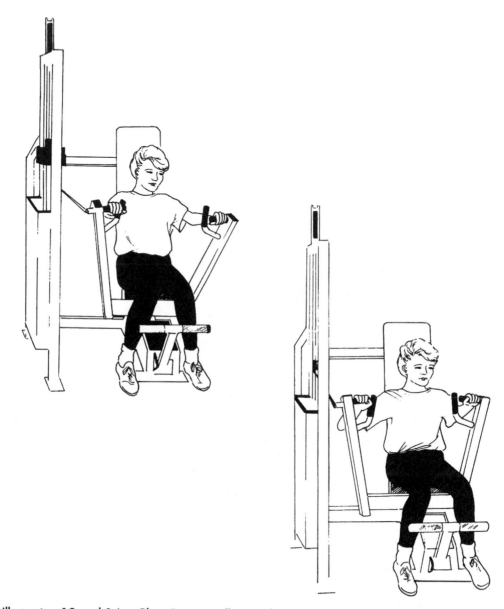

Illustration 13 and 14 – Chest Press – will strengthen arm bones and muscles.

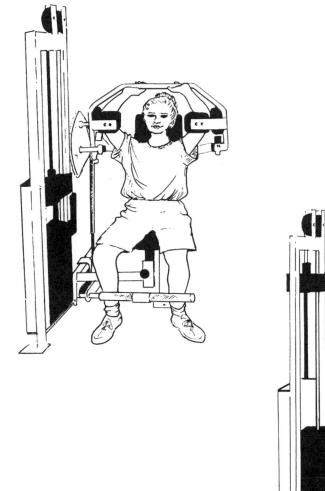
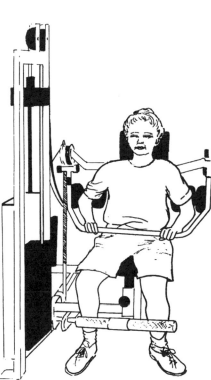

Illustration 15 and 16 – Rehabilitation, Pullover – strengthens wrists, abdomen and shoulders.

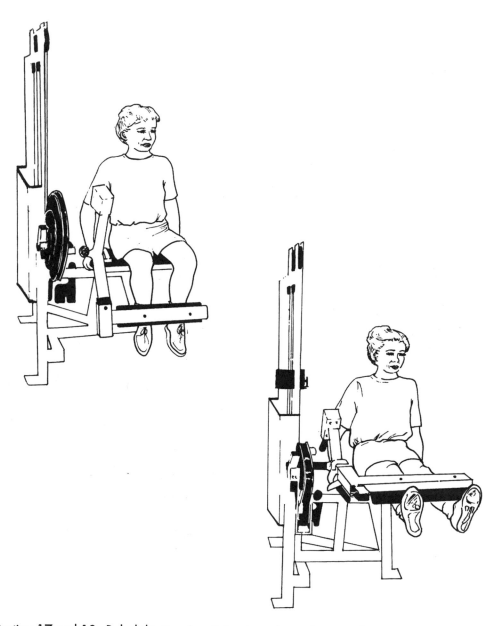

Illustration 17 and 18– Rehabilitation, Leg Extension – keeps femur or hip strong.

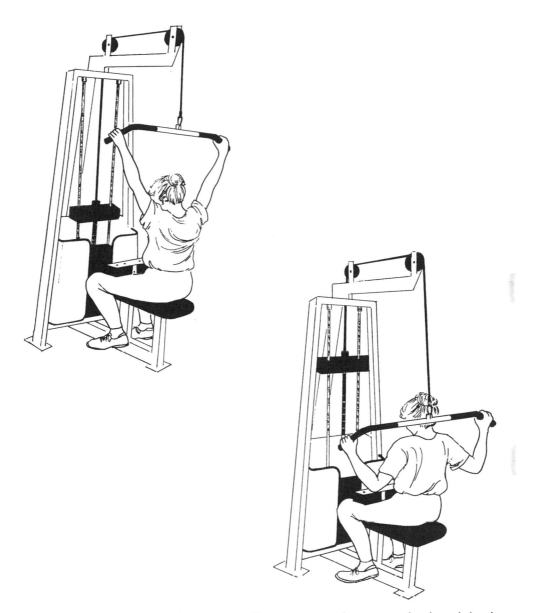

Illustrations 19 and 20 – Rehabilitation, Lat Pull Down – strengthens wrists, back and shoulders.

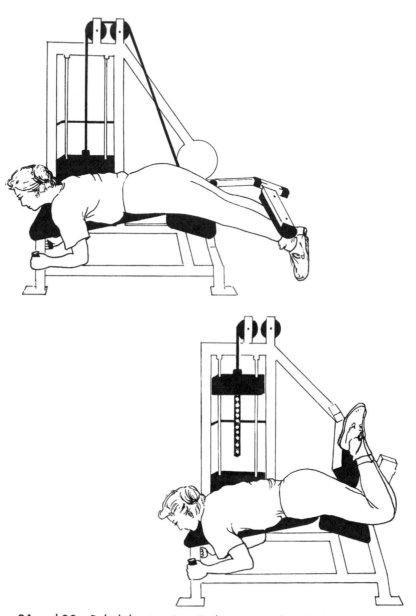

Illustrations 21 and 22 – Rehabilitation, Leg Curl – to strengthen the hamstring muscles and the femur or thigh and hip bone.

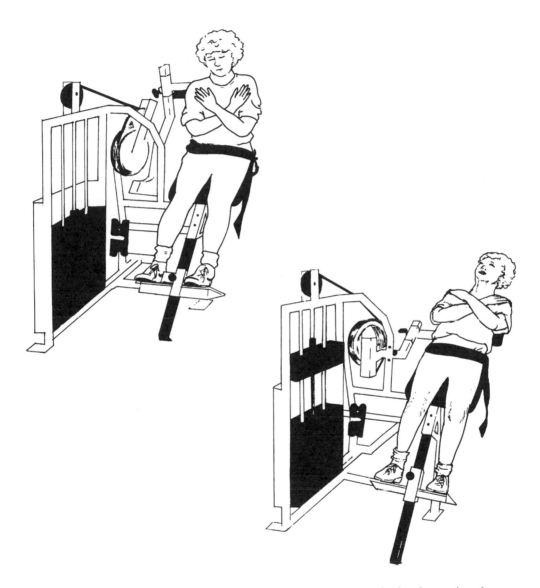

Illustration 23 – Rehabilitation, Back Strengthening – the stronger the back muscles, the stronger the vertebrae.

At 62, Beth was a white post-menopausal woman who early, at age 45, followed the menopause histories of her mother and sister. She had been sedentary for years, had arthritis, an ulcer, and diverticulitis (an inflammation of abnormal tubular sacks on the colon). She was an addicted smoker of 40 years. Her favorite activity was watching soap operas and living in dreams the lives of television stars.

Four vertebral fractures and crushing back pain caused Beth to seek help. Her bone density was significantly below average for her age. She took in about 1000 mg of calcium daily as well as estrogen for two years to arrest bone loss.

The Metamucil Beth was giving herself for her diverticulitis can bind oral estrogen tablets and her high fiber diet may have been binding the calcium she took. The aluminum-containing antacids for her ulcer probably bound up her calcium and helped to soften her bones.

She was willing to exercise if she could do it in front of the television, so we suggested she use a treadmill. By working up to two hours of daily treadmill walking to keep stress on the hip and leg bones, taking her calcium at a different time than her high-fiber breakfast, and saving one calcium dose to take at night (much calcium loss occurs at night) Beth began to show improvement. Her antacid was changed to a calcium-containing brand and her total daily intake of calcium was limited to about 1500 mg. Beth wanted to live without the threat of a hip fracture causing a shortened or crippled life.

The diagnostic tests for osteoporosis are three in number and are used to detect the state of bone health usually when you are between 35 and 50 years old. X-rays show osteoporosis but only when one-third of the bone density is already lost.

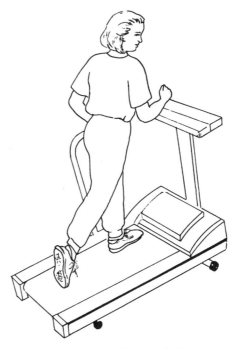

Illustration 25 – Treadmill – weight-bearing exercise for the hips.

— 28 —

You certainly don't want to wait for that to happen. But should an X-ray indicate that you have significant bone loss, you will want to start making changes in your life immediately. Since X-rays are not an accurate method to check for beginning osteoporosis, a highly technical apparatus called Quantitative Computed Tomography (QCT) is used (see Illustration #9, page 19). Scanning with this device tests the bones of the spine for signs of weakness. Scans of this nature are available in large medical centers. Dual Photon Absorptiometry (DPA) also shows bone weakness in the hip and spine. These tests quickly reveal whether or not you have adequate bone density. Dual Energy X-Ray Absorptiometry (DEXA) is more precise, but not available everywhere. Ask your doctor which tests are available in your community.

The DEXA scans measure bone density and should be repeated every one to two years in high-risk individuals. Your response to therapy can be monitored by the tests to gauge the effectiveness of the program you're following.

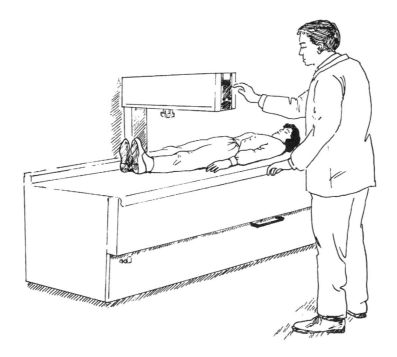

Illustration 26 – Dual Energy X-Ray Absorptiometry (DEXA).

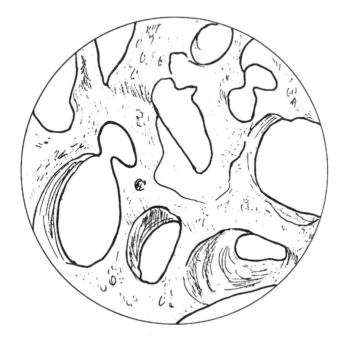

Illustration 27– Healthy Bone.

Osteoporosis is the most significant health hazard to the mature woman. The risk factors are older age, white race, early menopause, low calcium intake, physical inactivity, low body weight, smoking, excess alcohol and caffeine consumption. These are complicated by the binding of estrogen and calcium by medications aimed at treating other medical problems. Ask your doctor or dietitian for help in sorting out all the nutritional aspects of this problem.

You must become your own expert on osteoporosis. Design what you think should be an appropriate program of treatment using this book and present your plan to your health care provider. You'll feel like you have some control of your health again.

Remember, bones are living and ever-changing in the process of remodeling themselves. In a house, remodeling may mean removing a wall and replacing it with a counter or half-wall. Bones are busy constantly responding to stress by remodeling their lines of strength. See the pictures showing the strength lines of the hip on page 62.

Osteoblasts build bone while osteoclasts crunch or kill bones. Our bones are usually in harmony between the processes of building and tearing down. Without adequate stress placed on bones from exercise, the lines of strength gradually disappear. It's similar to what happens if you were to remove one 2x4 stud out of a wall of your house every few months. Eventually the wall could no longer stand. The same is true of the bones of the spine and hip. These stress lines need to be stimulated with exercise. IT IS NEVER TOO LATE TO START AN EXERCISE PROGRAM.

Armed with information and a desire to save your own life, you can take control of your own future. Request a bone density test at about age 50 or when you stop having periods to see if you are at high risk for osteoporosis due to low density bone.

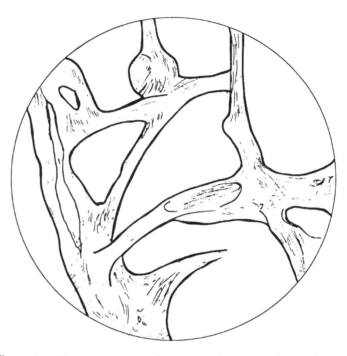

Illustration 28 – Osteoporotic bone; this illustration shows there is less of it.

... 3 ...

Calcium: How To Get It, How To Keep It

Calcium has been called "cowcium" by the American Dairy Association for good reason. Most dairy products have high amounts of calcium. See the chart on calcium content of foods in this chapter.

Bone can change remarkably in 10 years as is demonstrated on pages 30 and 31.. Bones act as a reservoir for calcium in the body. Calcium constantly is being taken from the bone storehouse to be used for muscle contraction and to help with enzyme systems in the body. Normally there is a perfect balance between calcium intake and calcium outflow through the urine after being used in the body. Osteoporosis is the result of calcium loss in excess of the amount ingested. What can you do?

The trick is knowing what foods are high in calcium and then figuring a way to get these into your diet. Some of these foods are also high in fat so you must be selective. With the graying of America, baby boomers of the 40s and 50s are reaching menopause. Osteoporosis will reach critical levels in this population. This is the first group to grow up in the shadow of the Barbie Doll without sufficient calcium, and we expect catastrophic problems from osteoporosis. To the baby boomers, dairy products, high in calcium, have lost some of their luster because of the calories.

High schools are serving skim, and chocolate milk to encourage teens to get adequate calcium. Parents are serving Manicotti stuffed with cheese; puddings are made with skim milk and low fat cheese sauces are filling the shelves in the grocery stores. Orange juice and cereals are fortified with calcium. Frozen yogurt shops have become ubiquitous. These substitutes for the calcium Americans once derived from milk are all beginnings of control of this devastating problem.

Thank goodness for magazines like Prevention, Shape, Runners World, Walking and Bicycling. They stress the joy of exercise while providing low-cal advertisements about many high-calcium foods. They give directions on how to manage your hectic life-style while taking care of your needs for physical exercise and nutrition.

Many of our patients' attitudes and philosophies have changed after reading the "success story" of an anorectic or bulimic personality who was able to gain pounds to reach her ideal weight. The opposite is also true. Obese, lethargic, constantly-tired women have started exercising, watching calories and paying attention to micronutrients including calcium.

The emphasis on health in the media, promoting lithe, flowing female bodies as the ideal of perfection, is helping to prevent complications of osteoporosis and the degenerative diseases like osteoarthritis. Antacid companies advertise in magazines and demonstrate how much calcium is available in their products.

Look at some of the high-calcium foods to see which ones you usually include in your diet. Here is a short list of the calcium content of certain foods. The selection of foods shown on the list was chosen for calcium qualities.

Food Item	Milligrams of Calcium
Almonds, 1/2 cup	100
Bagel	30
Beef, chicken in cheese sauce, 8oz	350
Bean burrito	200
Beans, 1 cup	100
Berries, 1 cup raw	40
Bok choy, 1 cup cooked	250
Bread, 1 slice	30
Broccoli, 1 cup	100
Buttermilk, 8oz	300

Food Item	Milligrams of Calcium
Carnation instant breakfast, 1 cup	400
Most cheeses, 1oz	200
Cheeseburger	150
Cheese pizza, 1 piece	100
Cream soups, 8oz	150
Cottage cheese, 8oz	150
Custard, 1 cup	300
Dandelion greens, 1 cup	300
Dates, 1 cup	100
Dry cereal with 1/2 cup milk	150-350
Egg	25
Fig bar	10
Ice cream, 1 cup	200
Ice milk, 1 cup	200
Kale, 1 cup	200
Orange juice with calcium, 8oz	200-300
Macaroni and cheese, 1 cup	200
Manicotti with cheese	300-500
Milkshake, 16oz (Use low fat products)	900
1% milk, 8oz	300
Skim milk, 8oz	300
Milk, nonfat, dry, 1 tblsp	100
Milk chocolate bar, 2oz	150
Muffin, English	100
Mushrooms, 1 cup	100
Mustard greens, 1 cup	200
Orange	60
Oysters, 1 cup	225
Pancakes, 4-inch made with milk	100
Peanuts, 1/2 cup	50
Peas, 1 cup	40
Puddings made with milk, 1 cup	200
Raisins, 1 cup	100

Food Item	Milligrams of Calcium
Rhubarb, 1 cup cooked	200
Rice, 1 cup	20
Roll, breakfast or Danish	25
Salmon, 3oz	200
Sardines, #8	400
Sherbet, 1 cup	100
Spinach, 1 cup	200
Shrimp, 3oz	100
Sweet potato, 1 med	50
Tofu, 1/4 cup	150
Tomato, 1 med	25
Tuna, 3oz canned	200
Waffle, 7inch	125
Walnuts, 1/2 cup	50
Frozen yogurt, 6oz	150
Yogurt, lowfat, 1 cup	400

If you haven't been reading labels regarding calcium content, start now. Keep the slender body if you want, but fill the bones with calcium.

Studies have shown that the bone density (how much calcium and protein there is in the bone) at the time of menopause will determine your risk for osteoporosis. If you have dense, strong bones at menopause, you will not be likely to suffer from osteoporotic fractures. Most of the bone mass growth occurs from age 10 to 20 years when bones are enlarging. After age twenty, the bones thicken which is why older people are thicker or heavier. Calcium can be added to the bones during the 20s, 30s, and 40s as the bones thicken. Preventing osteoporosis is easier than treating the problem. Make eating as enjoyable as you can by watching fats while making sure you get adequate calcium. Drink Vitamin D fortified milk unless you are outside in the sun for twenty or more minutes daily. The sun acting on the oils in your skin will make Vitamin D to help absorption of calcium.

Here is an easy way to read labels. A label from a container of skim milk is used as an example.

Nutrition Information Per Serving

Size ....1 cup
Servings per container 4
Calories 90
Protein 9%
Carbohydrates 12%
Fat 0

Percentage Of U.S. Recommended Daily Allowance (U.S. RDA)

Protein 20%	Vitamin D 25%
Vitamin A 10%	Vitamin B6 ....04%
Vitamin C 04%	Vitamin B12 ....15%
Thiamine 08%	Phosphorus...........25%
Riboflavin.............30%	Magnesium...........10%
Zinc......................06%	CALCIUM...........30%

One cup of skim milk provides 30% of the RDA of calcium. It takes 3-1/2 glasses of skim milk to meet the requirements for teens (1000 mg) and five glasses in a day to meet the extra needs during pregnancy or nursing. Older women require about 1500 mg daily. You needn't limit your calcium consumption to dairy products only, but keep them in mind for a good source of calcium.

How do you know if you are getting enough calcium? Use the list above or the list in any of the reference books to add up your total calcium intake for four days. Next, divide by four for your average daily intake of calcium. Are you getting enough? If not, use non-calorie TUMS or some other calcium supplement to make up the difference for your age requirements.

Total calcium intake for 4 days		_____ mg
Hidden calcium in other foods—	200 mg per day	_800 mg
	Total	_____ mg
Divide by 4 for daily calcium in milligrams		_____ mg

How much is enough? Premenopausal women need about 1000 mg daily. Postmenopausal, pregnant and nursing women need about 1500 mg daily. Earlier recommendations of less than 1000 mg may not be adequate. Some calcium supplements do not dissolve in the body and are worthless. Ask your pharmacist which calcium supplements work best.

There is also a home test to determine if your calcium is being absorbed. Put your calcium pill into a glass of white vinegar and let it stand for thirty minutes. If the pill doesn't dissolve in thirty minutes, it probably won't dissolve in the acid bath of your stomach and won't be helpful.

Supplement the calcium in your diet to meet your requirements as noted above. Now you have taken the first step towards keeping powerful bones from becoming powdery bones.

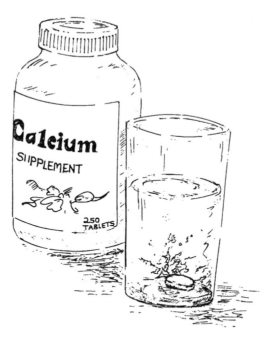

Illustration 29 – Dissolving Calcium in White Vinegar.

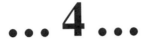

... 4 ...

What Is This Thing Called Menopause?

"I can't think straight any-more." Sheila whispered, with a bewildered expression on her face. She dropped the book she was reading in her lap. "I have a buzzing in my head," she said.

"What was that?" Asked her husband, Dan, from across the room.

"I must have been mumbling," she answered, not realizing she had spoken aloud.

Dan returned to his newspaper, ruffling the crisp pages like a reprimand for her interruption of his concentration. Sheila, a little frightened, tried to figure out what was happening to her. Her mind seemed to be working in

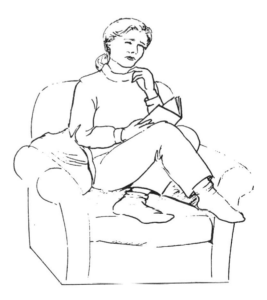

Illustration 30 – Sheila's Inability To Concentrate.

— 39 —

slow motion; she felt anxious because her thoughts seemed to be reduced to a terrifying crawl.

What is the matter with me? Why do I feel so on edge? Am I going crazy?

Sheila slipped back into her mystery book, but couldn't concentrate on Dirk Pitt, the hero of the story who was crawling in extremis across the desert in his quest to save the world from greedy businessmen.

Thousands of women like Shiela have experienced the self doubts and anguish that accompany menopause.

Stepping into menopause is like walking in front of a Mack truck. Women feel as if their bodies are falling apart. They suffer alone mostly with unanswered questions about what is happening to them.

Why the lack of information and help on the subject? Why the female taboo about speaking out on menopause and the anxious feelings that accompany it? Why don't women know what to expect?

Television shows the ideal female body full of youth, vigor and sexual attractiveness. The lovely woman portrayed on the screen maintains her popularity and beauty until the mid-thirties when she is slowly shuffled to the side stage by producers who replace her with a new youthful model. The older woman disappears for ten or fifteen years then shows up in a TV miniseries in a minor role as a mother of a teenage daughter. Menopause, a fact of nature, is ignored as if it were an inconvenience to be waited out until the affected woman regains her equilibrium — as if she were to blame for getting older.

Another reason that menopause was ignored for so long was due to coronary heart disease in men. Starting in the mid 1950s, they were dropping like flies from heart disease. Billions of dollars were spent on saving the "breadwinner" from this scourge. If a woman was suffering and struggling with menopause while her husband was having angina when going upstairs, her symptoms were swept away in the crisis of her spouse.

Women used to have a shorter life-expectancy and never experienced the post-menopause or its consequences for any length of time. In the early 1900s a woman was expected to live about 48 years. She died before menopause happened. Now, life is slightly more than half-started when women begin losing their femininity. Their breasts sag, their bodies stoop and their skin develops more lines than Rand-McNally. Irritability and frustration creep in and weakness seizes the muscles.

At a time when women are being freed from the responsibility of raising children, their bodies started to abandon them. Femininity has been associated with firm breasts, slender legs and hips and smooth, tight skin. Estrogen is responsible for these traits of women and its withdrawal signals tremendous changes in physical appearance. Flushing and gushing attack women at business meetings, in church, while playing golf or tennis, anytime. Unexpected, warm flowing blood has created a million excuses for women, forcing them to excuse themselves and back out of a room with a red spot growing on the back of their dress or slacks. Just as the first period for a woman may have come during junior high physical education class or at a dance, the first gusher of menopause may come about the time a woman turns 50.

But, talking about menopause has become ALMOST acceptable. You'll never hear a movie star admitting she is experiencing the menopause, which is interpreted as being synonymous with losing her youthful sex appeal. Menopause may be a natural part of life, but it is still shrouded in mystery.

The sleep cycle seems especially susceptible to the sneaky attacks of the menopause. The ping pong effects of estrogen in the female body bouncing from high to low results in hot flashes and night sweats. Millions of women go through the nightly ritual of flinging off the covers as they awake with their nightgowns drenched with perspiration, followed by chills from their wet bodies. It's no wonder that depressions, anxieties, and irritability are common. Night after night of interrupted sleep will bring the mightiest to their knees. The brain is having a "brown-out." and the results are decreased concentration, memory impairment, diminished energy and drive.

But this is usually just the beginning! As estrogen production from the ovaries decreases with age, more signs appear. The nighttime flashes sneak into the daytime hours. With little warning a woman's face, neck and chest may become beet-red as her body reacts to the low estrogen levels. Vaginal dryness ensues and sexual intercourse may become uncomfortable or downright painful. The skin of the vagina and the labia thins and as a result, the vagina may become very sensitive to infections or irritations. Urinary incontinence may develop. Estrogen helps protect women from heart disease but with its withdrawal at menopause, women develop the same rate of heart attacks as men. Women and heart disease have been ignored. Doctors thought women had permanent protection from heart disease due to estrogen.

How do you handle the menopause? What should you expect? What do you need to put up with?

When Sheila looked up from her book and announced to her husband, "Dan, I think I'm going through the change," she encountered the male antipathy to the menopausal symptoms of aging in women:

"What change?" Dan asked.

"You know, the change of life, the menopause," she said.

"Don't tell me you're going to turn into one of those witches I hear about at work with the tears and tantrums," he said accusingly.

Sheila was afraid to say anymore. If Dan wouldn't listen to her, who would?

Husbands are possibly the worst source for support and understanding during menopause. While they don't put it in so many words, they associate menopause with the loss of femininity, the onset of decrepitude. It is a threat to their perception of their mate as a desirable, youthful companion and lover. They don't understand and don't feel the changes their mates are going through. Doctors also can be a poor source of information with their hectic schedules. Many physicians don't research the literature on menopause and female doctors are often so busy they ignore their own symptoms. "I breezed through it," they may say. "You can too."

This short chapter is intended to give just a glimpse of the changes that occur with the menopause. If you want greater detail, I suggest you read one of the books on menopause in the recommended books section of your public library to understand the process more thoroughly.

What do you do when you are flushing and sweating at 3 a.m. and your heart is flip-flopping in your chest? You secretly sneak out of bed and walk out on the back porch. The thermometer by the window registers 35 degrees but your own thermostat is stuck on high. Sweat is running down your neck and your night clothes look like you've been playing basketball in the NBA. Thank goodness for the breeze. If your neighbors see you they probably wonder what possesses you to stand outside in near freezing weather in a skimpy nightgown.

Once the hot flash passes you feel suddenly chilly as the sweat has crusted and dried. You change clothes then get back into bed but the sheets are soaked so you cover them with a towel vowing to change them later before your husband notices.

Menopause can be difficult enough without some support from a female friend, but don't look to the friend for all the answers. She is searching for the same answers. Discovering from her that you aren't going crazy because you both have similar experiences is heartening.

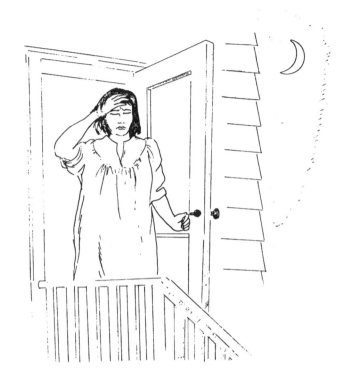

Illustration 31 – Woman Having Hot Flashes at Night.

If you haven't noticed signs of osteoporosis; bone pain, back pain, thin skin on the back of the hands, gum disease, or fatigue, then menopause will get your full attention as it flashes signals of bone changes.

Menopause is the beginning of an insidious attack on your bones. Holding back the log jam of unusual and unwanted feelings may take most of your energy, but don't let your bones dissolve while you are struggling with the life changes.

For one third of all women, menopause starts at the time of a hysterectomy which can be very premature for mother nature. The other two-thirds usually start between the ages of 48 and 55, with 50 being the average age in America. Since the aging process is one of life's mandatory events, what can we do to help overcome some of its less desirable results? Can estrogen help?

Estrogen is the processor for your central control center. It instructs hundreds of bodily functions how to work properly. It stops hot flashes, creates a sense of well being, stops bone loss, smooths out skin and restores the vaginal lining. It can help you to sleep better at night, function better during the day, and may even improve your sex life. Even the heart will benefit from its multitude of actions. Estrogen sounds like the next wonder drug and for some it is.

Sheila went to her gynecologist and he prescribed estrogen for her of 0.625 mg daily for 25 days each month and progesterone 5.0 mg daily for 10 days of each month. She felt great the first 15 days of the month when she took estrogen but from the 16th to the 25th of each month she took progesterone and felt terrible. The progesterone caused headaches, bloating, acne, nausea and irritability. One third of the month feeling like a basket case was too much for her. Back to her doctor she went for advice. He changed her estrogen dosage so that she took it every day and reduced her progesterone dosage by half to 2.5 mg daily. The drawback of the decreased progesterone dose was the longer interval of time that she had to take it. Fortunately, it worked. The smaller dose reduced the side affects to a tolerable level. She decided the estrogen- progesterone combination was worth taking for the clarity of mind it produced and because she felt like herself again.

Sheila's friend, Pam, wasn't as fortunate. Pam was going through the menopause but was still having sporadic periods. She felt confused, tired, irritable, had a loss of sex drive but most of all her job

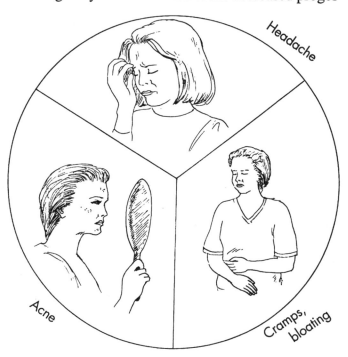

Illustration 32 – Side Effects of Progesterone.

as an accountant had suddenly become a nightmare. The figures and the forms became increasingly difficult and she moved more slowly. Her work took 10 hours a day instead of eight and she took work home at night to keep up.

After talking to Sheila, Pam visited with her doctor, had a physical, a pap test and an endometrial biopsy — a sampling of cells taken from inside the uterus for testing. The tests were fine and Pam was prescribed estrogen 0.625 for 25 days each month and progesterone 10 mg for 10 days each month.

Pam felt normal for 30 days, then developed leg pains the second month from phlebitis, an inflammation of the veins often caused by estrogen. The hormonal therapy had to be stopped. Depression set in as Pam thought she'd have to feel miserable for years. Fortunately, she sought out a nutritionist with an interest in hormonal remedies who recommended vitamin and mineral supplements, a change of diet without caffeine and refined sugar and a regular exercise program at a gym. See chapter 6.

Pam moved out of the smoky office she shared with another accountant, kept ice water with lemon slices for drinking in place of coffee and exercised aerobically every day. She felt more normal. She had a baseline Dual Photon Absorptiometry (DPA) test to check her bone density and planned on checking it in two years to be sure her life style changes were enough to keep her bones hard.

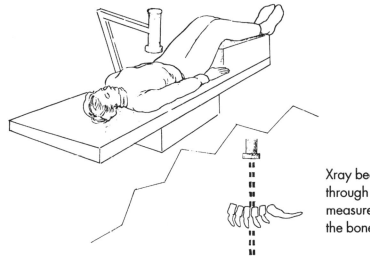

Xray beam passes through the bone to measure density of the bone.

Illustration 33 – Dual-Photon Absorptiometry (DPA).

Another woman, Nancy, did not want to keep having periods. "I'm tired of the monthly curse."

Nancy was a 50-year-old primate researcher with long days and evenings that stretched into the early morning hours in her attempt to track and record the life cycle and social strata of the chimpanzee. Her only outside activity was her five-mile run in the mornings to wake up and help keep her slender shape.

"For 38 years I've had periods and I'm sick of them," she said. Nancy had started menopause, actually the perimenopause, the time when the periods become irregular and unpredictable, but before the periods actually stop. She had experienced a few "gushers" and was disgusted that she had lost some of the control in her life. For years her periods had been predictable and she had been able to prepare for them. Her heavy episodes of vaginal bleeding characteristic of menopause were like going through adolescence all over again. Now she always carried tampons and pads "in case."

During her annual visit with her gynecologist, Nancy had spoken with the nurse and was advised that to prevent osteoporosis after the menopause, a combination of estrogen 0.625 mg and progesterone 2.5 mg could be taken every day of the month. After a few months, her periods would stop. She was glad for the advice and asked for the prescriptions.

"What a relief," she thought. "Finally my life is predictable again."

Hormone replacement therapy, HRT, as it is called, worked for Nancy, and can be a godsend but it isn't for everyone. Who should consider estrogen replacement therapy?

The Estrogen Dilemma

The whole question of hormone replacement therapy (HRT) has produced a controversy since some applications can produce cancer in women. Every woman should be aware of the facts of HRT and to that end the estrogen dilemma is treated in this chapter. Presented here is a brief summary of 30 years of HRT research which will give you a clearer understanding of estrogen replacement.

Hormone replacement therapy attempts to replace sex hormones, estrogen, progesterone, and sometimes testosterone, in those women who no longer produce sufficient quantities to meet the demands of their bodies.

Estrogen and progesterone are primarily produced by the follicles in the human female. A follicle is an egg that is surrounded by a special group of cells in the ovaries. At birth, a woman has approximately two million eggs. She will never produce any more, ever. By the time she reaches adolescence, the number of follicles in the female have decreased to about 300,000. It is from these follicles that all of her children will arise and it is from them that most of a woman's estrogen, progesterone and testosterone is produced. Each month some of the follicles are used up by the process of ovulation, or just by atrophy. In most women, there are only a few hundred follicles left as she approaches her mid-forties. When these are gone, menopause occurs. Thus, menopause is the condition that develops when the ovaries run out of eggs and estrogen and progesterone production falls.

After menopause, there is still a small amount of estrogen present, but much less than before menopause. This estrogen comes from chemicals produced in the adrenal glands — the small glands that sit on top of the kidneys. Fat cells help to convert the adrenal gland chemicals into estrogen. If the production of adrenal gland precursors is high or if a woman has a good proportion of body fat, then she may be able to breeze through menopause without all the unpleasant symptoms of menopause. She may avoid the hot flashes, night sweats, the vaginal irritation and dryness, the insomnia, headaches and the depression and irritability that happens to many women.

If the body doesn't produce estrogen on its own, then these symptoms develop, along with the silent dissolution of the bones — the dreaded signature of osteoporosis. By taking HRT, women not only hope to avoid these symptoms but also to prevent osteoporosis and heart disease. HRT effectively accomplishes these goals. But HRT involves risks as well as benefits. You must weigh the benefits and risks to make the best possible choice for yourself.

In the sixties, estrogen was the fifth most commonly prescribed medication, physicians prescribing it to avoid or soften the symptoms of menopause in their female patients. The risks of estrogen therapy weren't well known. Soon, however, it became apparent that there were drawbacks associated with estrogen replacement miracle drugs. By the mid- seventies a marked increase in endometrial (uterine) cancer was discovered in women who were taking estrogen replacements over a long term. About the same time, DES (diethylstilbesterol), another estrogen-like medication made the world news. This was a miracle pregnancy medication that supposedly prevented miscarriages as well as a number of other pregnancy complications. It was later found to promote the development of a very unusual cancer in the daughters of those women who took it during their pregnancy. Additionally, it caused some subtle changes in the reproductive tract of the babies exposed to the drug, leading to problems with infertility in today's generation of women. These cancer risks became a legacy of estrogen, and even today many women avoid any consideration of hormone replacement therapy for fear of developing cancer. Some advocates of doing away with hormone replacement therapy have been alarmist in their warnings of serious consequences for women who take hormone replacements.

Birth control pills, which had much higher doses of estrogen and progesterone than do the pills of today, were associated with strokes, heart attacks, liver disease and abnormal blood clotting. Some studies showed a link between long-term estrogen use and breast cancer.

Since those early days, much lower and safer dosages of estrogen and progesterone are found in birth control pills. These lower dosages of female hormones are effective in preventing pregnancy, but they are also effective in helping to prevent osteoporosis while reducing the risks of heart attacks, strokes and blood clots.

Presently, HRT involves a combination of low dose estrogen and progesterone that appears to significantly decrease the risk of heart disease, osteoporosis and endometrial cancer as well as to decrease the unpleasant menopause side affects. So then you may ask, *If HRT is so great, why do only 15-20% of women take this replacement therapy?*

The answer to this question is that realistic fears about potential side effects keep some women away from HRT while other women say that menopause is a natural transition in life and not a disease. These "naturalists" believe that HRT means adding a foreign substance to the body.

It is important for every woman to understand that HRT is hormone *replacement* therapy versus the idea of hormone *addition* therapy. As the human life span increases, women will spend one third of their lives in the postmenopause time period. This wasn't true in the past. Many physicians and patients believe that estrogen is essential for protection against osteoporosis and heart disease. How do you decide if HRT is for you?

HRT isn't for everyone. Each woman must make an individual decision whether in her case the benefits outweigh the risks. Social factors and past medical problems, along with your doctor's biases and opinions, enter into and complicate the picture. Be sure your decision is an informed one. Study the information in this chapter and then ask your doctor about HRT. Often your physician can provide you with informational videos and literature about menopause and hormone replacement. The pharmaceutical companies provide a wealth of patient information materials to doctors for patient education. Ask your doctor what materials he or she can provide you. Free magazine subscriptions are available from the major drug companies, and they are available to you just for the asking. Check with your doctor for details. A physician's office with a paucity of information on menopause and HRT, or a physician who won't take the time to answer your questions, obviously may not have an interest in this phase of life so you may have to choose another physician or be assertive and seek information at libraries or bookstores. Remember, information is the key to knowledge and as American novelist Ethel Mimford once said, "Knowledge is Power."

The days are gone when a woman with hot flashes, night sweats and irritability is immediately given a prescription for estrogen only. Today, progesterone, the hormone produced during the second half of the menstrual cycle, is typically added to the estrogen replacement therapy. Because of the uterine cancer scares of the 1970s from estrogen replacement there have been some excellent studies completed that show that if progesterone is replaced along with estrogen, then the risk of endometrial cancer can be reduced to zero.

Which type of estrogen is best? The natural human estrogens are estradiol, estrone, and estriol. Estrogen replacement therapy includes one or more of these substances or compounds and are chemically very similar to the natural forms. They are artificially produced in the lab, derived from plant materials, or obtained from animal products. Birth control pills have higher levels of synthetic hormones because higher doses of estrogen are necessary to prevent ovulation. Therefore, birth control pills or oral contraceptives can have more side effects than the estrogens which are prescribed for menopause symptoms. Oral contraceptives are usually not prescribed after menopause as there is no need to prevent ovulation and the side effect profile is unwarranted after menopause.

The most commonly used estrogen preparation is Premarin (pre-mar-in), a mixture of naturally occurring estrogens derived from the urine of pregnant mares. It is frequently called a conjugated estrogen because of the many estrogens involved. Estradiol, the body's most potent form of estrogen, is the main component of Estrace and transdermal patches. Ogen is a derivative of estrone, a weaker form of estrogen produced by the ovaries and also by the conversion of androgen (male hormone) to estrogen by fat cells.

Is oral estrogen better than estrogen patches? Estrogen is usually taken in pill form once daily. Since we are all different, some women do not absorb enough estrogen this way to control their menopausal symptoms. When taken orally, the estrogen must pass through the liver before it reaches the blood stream. This has both good and bad points. The good points are that the pill form of estrogen replacement raises the HDL or high density lipoproteins which help to protect the woman from heart disease. The down side is that a woman with liver disease, gall bladder disease or with a history of blood clotting, the pill form may aggravate or worsen these problems. Also, some women have very sensitive stomachs when it comes to taking hormones. Nausea or indigestion can occur if pills are taken on an empty stomach. Lastly, pills tend to be less expensive than the transdermal patches.

The estrogen patches applied to the hip, thigh or abdomen twice a week will produce a steady level of estrogen as it is absorbed through your skin. This estrogen does not raise the HDL or good cholesterol, but it acts to lower the LDL (low density lipoprotein), or bad cholesterol and helps provide a good overall lipid profile. While the concept of never having to remember to take a pill is often appealing, what is often overlooked is that currently there is not a progesterone patch available on the market. That makes the question of choice academic and you would still have to take a progesterone pill to protect the uterus from endometrial cancer. Also, many women become sensitive to the adhesive which is used to hold the patch on the skin. A rash or itching often means that you will have to switch to another, non-dermal form of estrogen. Some women have successfully pretreated the skin site with cortisone cream the day before the patch application if they are sensitive to the patch.

Injections containing one or more of the estrogen components may be used in women who do not absorb estrogen or who do not tolerate the patch due to persistent irritation at the site of application.

Women with a uterus intact who take estrogen should also take progesterone. Progesterone protects the uterus from endometrial cancer development. Progesterone helps nourish the egg and maintains the pregnancy should conception occur. If fertilization of the egg by sperm does not occur, then falling progesterone levels cause break down of the uterine lining. The endometrial cells are flushed out of the body, thereby completing the menstrual cycle with a normal period.

If progesterone is not produced or is not replaced during the cycle, then the uterine lining continues to grow in an unchecked fashion. Over a period of months, this uterine lining can become abnormally thickened, a condition called hyperplasia. The hyperplasia can persist for months to years, unbeknownst to the woman, and this is thought to be one of the mechanisms by which endometrial cancer develops.

Progesterone can be found as a naturally occurring substance or as a synthetic hormone. Synthetic progestins are usually stronger than their natural counterparts and are often the progestin component of oral contraceptives as well as the progesterone used in hormone replacement therapy. Medroxyprogesterone acetate is the generic name of the most common progesterone used in hormone replacement therapies. Some common names of medroxyprogesterone are Provera, Amen and Cycrin. Other synthetic progesterones are Norethindrone, Norgestrel and Levonorgestrel.

The natural progesterones are found in either suppository form or as an injectable in an oil-based solution. The compounds are often used for infertility work when you don't want an early embryo or fetus to be exposed to synthetic hormones.

So how much estrogen and progesterone are needed to prevent the symptoms of menopause, keep bones hard and yet avoid hyperplasia? When it comes to HRT, less is best … at least up to a point. In the past many women were started on high doses of conjugated estrogen because it wasn't known how much was necessary. Now, doctors are provided with guidelines on the minimum estrogen necessary to protect women without unnecessary risk from other complications. Recommended minimum doses of estrogen are 0.625mg of conjugated or esterified estrogens, 1 mg. of micronized estrogen, and 0.05 mg. of transdermal estrogen. Lower doses than these may control menopausal symptoms but will not protect against osteoporosis or heart disease. You will need to discuss this with your health care provider.

Progesterone doses are also varied depending upon the medication used and the preferences of the prescribing physician. Common doses of Provera range from 2.5 to 10 mg., with the lower doses prescribed for longer duration during any given month. Norethindrone doses range from 0.3 to 5 mg. per day while the natural progesterones usually range from 25 to 100 mg. per day.

Cycling to Mimic the Natural Menstrual Cycle
Many women choose to take HRT to simulate the normal cycle. They take conjugated estrogen 0.625mg for 25 days per month and start taking progestin in 5 to

10 mg doses from day 13 to 25 each month or cycle. You can just about count on having a period using this method of HRT because this regimen mimics the ovaries so well that the uterus is just doing what it thinks it is supposed to do … what it's been doing for the past 40 years, having a period. This last point is considered to be a major drawback of this regimen. Most women are happy to forever forsake the monthly curse of the period.

If you use the estrogen patch, the 0.05mg patch is similar in dosage to the 0.625mg conjugated estrogen while the 0.10 patch equals about 1.0 to 1.25mg of conjugated estrogen. Patches need to be changed twice weekly. This is nice because you don't have to remember to take a pill every day. Very athletic women sometimes have problems with the patch because it can come loose as they sweat. Also, some women are sensitive to the sticky glue which attaches it to your skin.

Many women find it unacceptable to continue having periods once the menopause has begun and a new Combined Continuous Regimen has become useful and popular. This program prevents build of the endometrium (hyperplasia) while preventing uterine bleeding. Often, initially, there is some spotting or breakthrough bleeding but this usually subsides after a few months.

What Are the Side Effects of HRT?

With most medications there are side effects. If you look at the list of side effects printed on an insert in an estrogen package, you'll find the warnings as long as your arm. Remember though, that many of these side effects were found using older estrogens at much higher doses than today's medicines. The most common side effect of women taking HRT is fluid retention, which can be translated into weight gain. "Eeek," you say! "After working hard to keep the pounds off, now you're telling me that this wonderful hormone will also add more weight to my already stressed body."

Well, yes. The fact is that estrogen rejuvenates many things in the body. Many enzymes are accelerated but the weight-producing culprit is angiotensinogen. This enzyme stimulates the production of renin which causes water retention. Reducing salt and caffeine along with regular exercise seems to combat this problem for many women, however, some women will need an occasional diuretic (water pill) to remove excess fluid.

Breast tenderness from estrogen acting on receptors in the breast tissue is an annoying side effect. The hormones stimulate the glands in the breasts to "plump up" to premenopausal levels. As they "plump," the breasts pull on the suspensory ligaments and this can result in breast tenderness. Sometimes making adjustments in the dosages of estrogen and progesterone will help. Usually, though, this goes away after a couple of cycles.

Migraine headaches are worsened in some women and are improved in others. One thing is sure though, if migraine headaches arise after starting HRT, most women will stop the treatment. The headaches may happen because of changes in hormone levels, so a steady dosing regimen such as the Combined Continuous method may work the best for these individuals.

How Should You Monitor the Consequences of HRT?

HRT is a "forever" adventure. You can indefinitely postpone all of menopause's unpleasantries as long as you continually provide the hormone that your ovaries used to make. Once the hormones stop, however, then so stops the protection that these hormones provide.

Estrogen affects the liver, heart, uterus, ovaries bladder, brain, skin and breasts as well as the thickness and moisture of other mucous membranes. At least yearly, you should have a Pap smear and pelvic exam along with a breast exam and mammogram.

Hospitals are now required by Medicare to send yearly reminder notes to patients who have had at least one mammogram in their X-ray department. Medicare has been trying to cut costs, but the medical directors at Medicare recognize the need for annual evaluation.

It must be emphasized that the risk of endometrial cancer is high if Hormone Replacement Therapy does not include progesterone. This is called unopposed estrogen stimulation and as I mentioned, it causes thickening (endometrial hyperplasia) of the uterine lining. The addition of progesterone to the estrogen therapy appears to counteract this effect. A 10-day supply of progesterone significantly reduces the risk of endometrial cancer and a 14-day progesterone regimen each month seems to completely eliminate the risk of endometrial cancer associated with estrogen replacement.

The risk factors associated with endometrial cancer can be summed-up as follows: The typical woman at risk for endometrial cancer is post- menopausal and obese with high blood pressure. She has typically never been pregnant or never carried a pregnancy to full term, and has infrequent periods.

Breast cancer has become a hot topic in America. In 1991, the news media flooded our consciousness with the results of a study which was published in the Journal of the American Medical Association stating that Estrogen Replacement Therapy (ERT) increased the risk of breast cancer. (The media ignored three earlier studies which showed no increased risk.) This launched a very close scrutiny of all the data done over the past 10-20 years to see if there was a genuine risk of breast cancer from our wonder drug, estrogen. The smoke hasn't settled on this issue yet, but many things are clearer. Breast cancer is the most common malignancy in the United States. Early "sensationalized" data quoted a woman's risk of developing breast cancer as one in nine. We now know that this high degree of risk is not seen until age 85. The risk at age 45 is one in 93. Who is especially at risk of breast cancer? The American Cancer Society publishes a list of risk factors, and as of April 1994, these are:

• Increasing age: The disease of breast cancer is rare in women under the age of 30; the incidence rises sharply in the 40s; levels off around 45; and then increases again after age 55.

• Family history; Women whose mothers or sisters have had breast cancer are two to three times more likely to develop breast cancer; the risk is even greater if these relatives have had cancer in both breasts or developed it before menopause.

• Previous breast cancer: 10-15% of women who have had cancer in one breast will eventually have it in the other.

• Diet: A high-fat diet has been linked to an increased risk, although this needs to be proven by upcoming clinical trials.

• Race or national origin: Breast cancer is more common among women of North American or Northern European origin than among women in Asian and African countries.

• Menstrual history: A long menstrual history - early onset of menstruation plus late menopause - increases the risk, while early menopause, either natural or artificial, decreases the risk.

• Pregnancy: The risk is higher among women who have never had a baby or whose first full-term pregnancy occurred after the age of 30.

• Hormonal factors: The relationship of hormones to breast cancer is unclear. Studies into a possible link between breast cancer and oral contraceptives have widely contradictory results. As with oral contraceptives, a link between estrogen replacement therapy and breast cancer is suspected by some scientists, but has not been proven.

• Some benign, proliferative changes seen in breast biopsy specimens are associated with an increased risk for subsequent development of breast cancer.

• Factors which do not seem to increase the risk of breast cancer: 1) an injury to the breast, 2) sexual stimulation, and 3) breast feeding.

So, estrogen therapy may increase the risk of breast cancers in certain women. Did you notice that I said, "may?" Well, that's because it is so controversial right now. Many, many studies do not find any risk of breast cancer associated with HRT. Many, many studies do suggest a risk. If you could count the number of studies both for and against, you would probably find that the groups saying that there *is* a risk of breast cancer would win by a slim margin.

So the best answer right now about whether HRT raises the risk of breast cancer is, "we just don't know." If there is an increased risk, it will probably be small, but nevertheless it is something to keep an eye on as more data becomes available.

Magazine articles abound about the pros and cons of HRT, ERT, and breast cancer. Remember that highly sensationalized articles which discuss the dreaded affects of hormones will almost certainly sell better than those stories showing no adverse affect. Ask questions of your health care provider or others knowledgeable on the subject to get the whole picture or the latest statistics.

What about women who have already had breast cancer? If you have had breast cancer that was susceptible to estrogen stimulation then under no circumstances should you take estrogen for the time being. Several studies suggest the HRT will not cause a relapse of breast cancer but the data is far too new to test yet. One day the answer will be much clearer, but for now, don't take HRT if you have had breast cancer. Tests for estrogen receptors are performed on the breast tissue at the time of breast removal. This may be important information in the future if certain types of breast cancer patients are found to be safe to take estrogen. If you have had breast cancer, consult with a cancer specialist before even considering estrogen replacement therapy. Dr. A. Hadjipavlou M.D. in his classic chapter on *Osteoporosis Of The Spine And Its Management,* addresses the frequency of breast cancer in the population by stating "…that even a slightly increased risk, especially if hormone replacement therapy is prescribed for longer than 15 years is worrisome."

Heart attacks and strokes are a concern of women who take birth control pills. The author has seen women 30 years old in a nursing home with a stroke and paralysis from taking birth control pills, although, these were the older, higher dose pills.

Birth control pills contain higher dosages of estrogen or stronger estrogen than the estrogen prescribed at menopause. Older sources say that HRT should be avoided in women who have had blood clots or thrombophlebitis (a clot with vein inflammation), but in actuality, the risk is not fully known. Be cautious if you fall into this category. There does not appear to be any significant affect on blood clotting factors, but this doesn't describe the whole picture when discussing blood clotting.

The frequency of heart attacks with the lower doses of conjugated estrogen at menopause is less than that seen in the general population. Conjugated estrogen appears to improve the blood lipid profile and help prevent heart attacks.

The risks of HRT may be seen as too high a price to pay for hard bones, soft skin and control of hot flashes. Behind the scenes though, hip fractures from osteoporosis fill nursing homes every year and heart attacks end or change many women's lives. Do HRT benefits outweigh the risks?

The Journal of the American Medical Association in 1983 studied 2300 estrogen-using women for six years and found a lower incidence of death than in non-estrogen users. As mentioned earlier, osteoporosis and heart disease are more common than either breast or endometrial cancer. Heart attacks occur 14 times more often than endometrial cancer occurs. Many physicians feel that estrogen and progesterone affect the bones and small blood vessels and may add several years of health to the post-menopausal woman.

Menopause can be annoying and uncomfortable but the feelings are not life threatening. Osteoporosis and heart disease *are* life threatening. They silently stalk and strike when you least expect it. HRT can prevent or slow the development of heart disease and osteoporosis. Your decision to take HRT is a personal one. The risks of HRT may seem overwhelming. Why should you increase your chances of cancer or stroke to prevent hot flashes or mood swings? For many women who are not high risk for cancer, HRT provides benefits that outweigh the risks.

If you have a family history of osteoporosis, if you are thin or have light skin, if you have a family history of heart disease, if you had your ovaries removed before age 45, if you went through natural menopause before age 45, if you have uncontrolled hot flashes, vaginal dryness and discomfort, loss of energy, libido or lack of concentration, then consider hormone replacement therapy.

Who should worry about taking HRT? Do you have a family history of endometrial cancer or breast cancer that is sensitive to estrogen? Have you had episodes of unexplained uterine bleeding, do you have a history of blood clots, migraine headaches or phlebitis? If you answered yes to any of these questions, estrogen replacement therapy may not be for you. Research shows that if you take estrogen supplements for fifteen years or longer, you may increase your chances of getting breast cancer.

Estrogen is the elixir of youth for some and hemlock for others. In the proper setting, estrogen can literally be a life saver, but if you are at high risk of feminine cancers then think a second time. Have yearly pap smears and mammography of your breasts. Prevent problems.

If you can't take estrogen then you will need to make major modifications to your lifestyle and check your bone density periodically to keep the silent stalker, osteoporosis, at bay.

Talk to your health care provider about the side effects of any medication you take. Ask your local library for information. All the answers about hormone therapy are not in but the more information you have, the more informed will be your decision of whether or not to take Hormone Replacement Therapy.

Also, don't be tricked into feeling secure about breast cancer prevention because you are taking Tamoxifen, a medication that decreases breast cancer recurrence. Many doctors prescribe it to prevent any recurrence of breast cancer, but current literature shows that women who use Tamoxifen to prevent breast cancer have a two times higher risk of developing endometrial cancer. Any time hormones are manipulated in the body for any length of time, there is a chance of significant side effects. Many of the side effects are not totally known or understood at this writing. Make an informed decision. Read, study and talk with your health care provider. Remember, "knowledge is power."

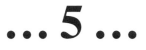

... 5 ...

Is There Life After A Hip Fracture?
Don't Despair!

Spine crush fractures usually heal without surgery, but hip fractures require some type of surgery for recovery. If your hip breaks is that the beginning of the end? Absolutely not!

Never take a hip fracture lying down. Bounce back. After surgery and a short hospitalization you'll usually be transferred to an extended care facility where rehabilitation begins. Rehabilitation means restoring the lost strength, flexibility, endurance and balance or neuromuscular coordination to your body. With effort you can be in better physical condition after surgery than you were before.

Rehabilitation is not completed in the extended care facility, it is only a beginning to get you back home again, on your feet and able to take care of yourself. It represents minimal rehabilitation. The rehabilitation machines start with very light weights as opposed to the weights in a gym. Some of the machines use weights as light as four pounds compared to gym weights of twelve pounds or more.

Let's look as the case of a woman who fractured her hip.

Betsy, 64, fell as she stood up to get out of bed. A little dizzy after arising from her night's sleep, she lost her sense of orientation and fell. Her osteoporotic hip fractured as she crashed to the floor. She was in terrible pain. See illustration 34. She hurt too much to crawl to the phone and passed in and out of awareness due to the pain.

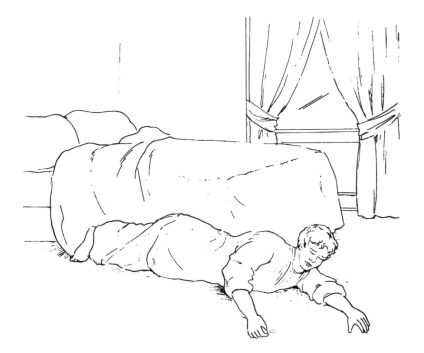

Illustration 34 – Betsy Fell as She Got Out of Bed.

Eight hours later her daughter called. Betsy heard the phone as if in a mist, but couldn't move. Her daughter came by to find the house door locked. She entered the house, found Betsy and called 911. The emergency crew gently placed Betsy on a stretcher as they protected her hip from movement.

Surgery was accomplished - a hip pinning. After a few days Betsy was transferred to a skilled nursing facility for daily physical therapy and for help with her living activities while she recuperated. She needed aid with dressing, bathing, cooking, the basic necessities of an independent life.

After three weeks of therapy, Betsy was able to live alone again but she was constantly in fear that she would break the other hip. She continued outpatient rehabilitation for three more weeks, taking a taxi from her home.

After a total of six weeks of therapy she was able to drive. The rehab clinic

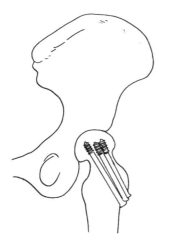

Illustration 35 – Pinned Hip.

allowed her to continue to participate in an independent program under supervision for about the same cost as a regular health club.

Betsy wanted to travel to see her grandchildren and watch them play sports so she determined she would work in the rehab unit to fully return her strength. She used the Cybex machines, the treadmill and the bicycle to accomplish her goal. See Chapter Two. After the rehabilitation she felt stronger and better than she had in years. She took daily calcitonin injections to help harden her bones.

Sometimes it takes an injury to remind people of the necessity to keep themselves strong and supple.

Research shows that weight bearing stimulates bone growth but, weight bearing plus aerobic activity produces more bone growth. Over a year's time calcitonin (an injectable thyroid hormone) increases calcium uptake and hardens the bone by eight percent in most women as measured by DPA-Dual Photon Absorptiometry.

Betsy realized how she'd let herself deteriorate prior to her hip fracture. "I'm going to make a new life," she vowed as she pulled on her Rockport walking shoes for a daily one hour walk. Never mind that the rains in Oregon where she lived were pounding the sidewalks, Betsy walked every day with her umbrella, her non-slip walking shoes and wrist weights to increase the weight on her hips.

Figures 36 through 38 show the gradual loss of bone strength lines that occur with inactivity, an excess of cortisone, Dilantin or excess thyroid supplement. The reverse is also true. You can restore some but not all of the strength lines in the non-surgical hip with effort and exercise.

What can you expect to be able to do after you've had a hip fracture? The answer can be positive if you take positive steps to renew your bones and strength. If you were in relatively good health and physical condition prior to your hip fracture, you have a good chance of returning to an active life. There is no reason to live as a couch potato. You can walk, swim, bicycle, play golf or tennis doubles, bowl or par-

Normal Bone   Moderately Weak Bone   Extremely Weak Bone

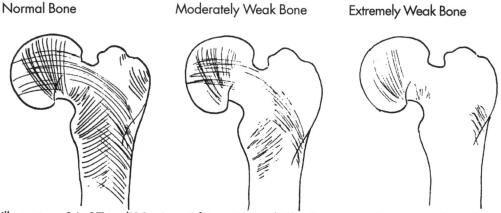

Illustrations 36, 37 and 38 – Loss Of Bone Strength. The illustrations demonstrate loss of force as strength lines decrease.

ticipate in any non-pounding activity. All the more reason to participate in seniorobics, chairobics or any kind of aerobic activity. Chairobics are performed sitting on a chair and pedaling a stationary bicycle from the back. See page 62.

Seniorobics are performed at a senior center in an exercise group.

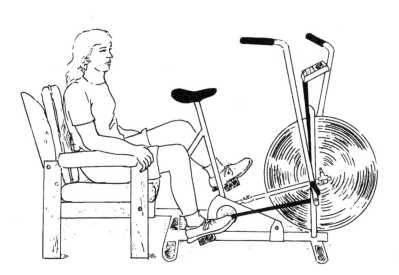

Illustration 39 – Chairobics.

As I've noted, calcitonin injections daily increase bone mass by an average of eight percent in the first year. Exercise adds to the bone mass as do calcium and Vitamin D. Wrist weights put extra stress (weight) on the hip joints to stimulate bone growth.

In another broken hip case,

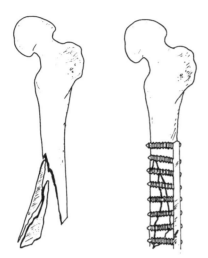

Illustration 40 – Hip Broken in the Long Shaft.

51-year-old Rebecca lived in a mobile home court with delightful neighbors who all cared about one another. Stepping out the front door of her home, she slipped on ice, fell and broke her hip in the long shaft. She had had a hysterectomy at age 40 for excessive bleeding but refused medications because she believed only in natural treatments.

After hip surgery she began therapy with assisted walking, then used a walker and finally graduated to a cane. Rebecca wanted to "toughen up her bones," so she read all the books at the library on natural treatments for osteoporosis. She took "natural substances", herbs vitamins and minerals including calcium. She took evening primrose oil which some people say acts like a natural estrogen.

DEXA X-ray testing showed her bone mass was slightly low for her age. Her healthy lifestyle prior to the injury had helped protect her bones but sometimes a direct fall on the hip will break any bone.

Rebecca's neighbors helped her until she could care for herself. She used a ski machine twice daily to strengthen her bones and muscles. A repeat DEXA scan a year later showed no change. No loss of additional bone mass was discovered, proving her program worked, so she dismissed her doctors and went her own way comfortable in her decision.

Bones respond to the stress placed on them. The two hours per day of practice skiing helped Rebecca's bones stay hard. Her focus on natural therapy with avoidance of caffeine, alcohol and smoke was an excellent example of taking charge of her life. Rebecca was given all the available options and successfully chose the ones that fit her beliefs and lifestyle.

What Do I Need to Know about Hip Fracture?

The older population has a commonly shared fear of a fractured hip. This injury is synonymous with social death if not real death. Your life may be forever changed if it happens to you. One common question about hip fractures requires an answer: Is it true or false that the hip breaks, after which the person falls? This is sometimes true, but usually the fall occurs on one side or the other of the hip, with a direct fall on one of the hip bones responsible for causing the fracture. At about age 60 we begin to lose the reflexes that help us catch ourselves if we fall. In addition, women's bones are softer than men's bones. Men fall frequently but their harder bones fracture less often.

What Can I Do to Avoid a Hip Fracture?

Keep taking the recommended doses of calcium, exercise regularly to stress your bones and to help with balance. Avoid smoke and excess alcohol and caffeine. Consider estrogen therapy if you are at high risk for fractures. Iowa State University has done a study using hip protectors on frail nursing home clients. These padded garments decreased hip fractures significantly. We can't all dress like football players with six pounds of pads on our bodies but hip pads could be a life saver for high-risk people when worn in the nursing home where many fractures occur.

One third of a million hip fractures will occur this year and more will be added to that number each year as the population grows older. You're hoping it won't happen to you and I hope you're spared this distressing problem. Hip fractures take an emotional toll on the patient and her family. Medical costs this year will be about $12 billion for hip fractures and secondary nursing home care. In five years the annual cost is estimated to rise to about $30 billion. Who pays for this expense, the insurance companies? They may write the checks but the costs are passed on to all of us. Your paycheck is shorted by more dollars every year for health care costs. We not only have a health care crisis, we have a HEALTH CRISIS in this country. We need better health.

Bones are strong and lightweight and designed to be used. Note the strength lines in the hip bone. See page 62. If not used, the lines vanish and with them goes the bone strength. Bike for your bones; work the muscles across the hip joint, step up to better health with a step machine. Pick a weight-bearing activity and start living again.

Safety in the Home

Home sweet home is the place we want to be especially as we age. As we spend more time at home we're less careful with our activities because we are so comfortable with the familiar surroundings. Bathtubs and showers can be a nightmare

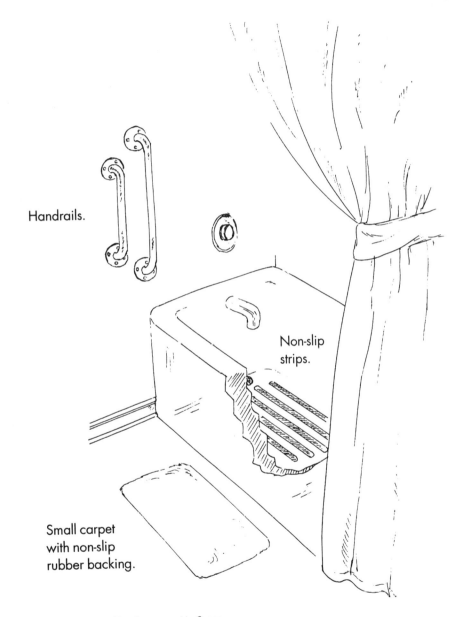

Handrails.

Non-slip
strips.

Small carpet
with non-slip
rubber backing.

Illustration 41 – Bathroom Safety.

unless you have bathtub strips or a rubber mat. If you are a little unsteady, put up a safety bar by the tub.

Keep a floor light on at night for frequent trips to the bathroom that are an indication of getting older. When you get out of bed, first sit on the edge of the bed for a few seconds to allow your blood pressure to adjust. Stand slowly and stay in place for two to three seconds then walk. Your blood vessels adjust more slowly to position changes after fifty especially if you are taking blood pressure medications, tranquilizers, or antidepressants.

Floors; get rid of throw rugs before they throw you. Don't polish floors, they become too slippery. Avoid walking on vinyl floors in socks because of slippage. Watch for uneven floors as your home ages. Move loose cords away from areas where you walk.

When using stairs, always use the rails for extra balance. With age 45 come bifocals and not quite as clear a focus as we look down, so keep items off the stairs and the floors. Safety in the home can save your hips and your life. Keep alert for obstacles and clutter. Prevent problems. An ounce of prevention ...

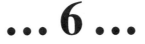

... 6 ...

Gym Exercise Stage 1 and Stage 2 Treatment

It's so easy not to exercise, to put off the exertion required until later. This procrastinating behavior is typical of thousand of Americans, but I wish to emphasize that women have but one choice: Exercise and stay healthy, or refrain and doom yourself to weak bones that can break with normal physical stress. I am sorry I have to be so blunt, but most of us are lazy when we contemplate working up a sweat. The strange part about exercise is that once you start, it becomes enjoyable and after a refreshing shower, your body actually glows with vigor. You feel better, energetic, full of zip.

William James wrote a small commentary on exercise that I think is worth printing here. It tells us that resistance to exercise did not start with our generation:

"Keep the faculty of effort alive in you by a little gratuitous exercise every day. That is, be systematically ascetic or heroic in little unnecessary points, do every day or two something for no other reason than that you would rather not do it, so that when the hour of dire need draws nigh, it may find you not unnerved and untrained to stand the test."

Well, the test for women comes when you reach an age — 50 to 65 — that makes you vulnerable to the disease that insidiously robs you of your stamina, vitality and resistance. You may not know your bones are sick until one of them fails. That's the time when "the hour of dire need" has drawn nigh. But if you will agree to discipline your life just a little, you never need to be "unnerved and untrained."

I think it's worthwhile to discuss briefly how exercise benefits women in particular. Today, only about six to eight percent of our population exercises adequately to preserve their vitality throughout their lifetimes. But what is the direct benefit of regular exercise? Individuals who exercise regularly enjoy better functional capacity. You probably will live longer, too, but more importantly you may live more years independently and postpone or entirely eliminate the need for family or institutional care.

Exercise is the central ingredient of good health. It tones the muscles, strengthens the bones, makes the heart and lungs work better, and helps prevent constipation. It increases physical reserve and vitality. The increased reserve function helps you deal with crises. Exercise eases depression, aids sleep, and enhances every activity of daily life.

It is well proven that physically fit women die from cancer 16 time less often than unfit women, and men and women who are fit are eight times less likely to die from cardiovascular disease.

Regular exercise helps reduce blood pressure and levels of harmful LDL cholesterol, while increasing the beneficial HDL cholesterol. Women who are physically active into older age are less likely to develop osteoporosis, and physically fit women are 33 percent less likely to get diabetes than unfit women.

These are impressive figures, pointing out that the benefits far out weigh the inconvenience.

You are never too old to begin an aerobic exercise program and to experience the often dramatic benefits. Always start slowly and build up slowly. Those who do too much too soon are the ones that get into trouble. You should be able to carry on a conversation while you are exercising. On the other hand, you should be breaking sweat during each exercise period if the exercise is performed at normal temperatures of approximately 70 degrees. The sweating indicates that the exercise has raised your internal temperature.

You need an exercise goal of 200 minutes per week spread over five to seven sessions; beyond this amount no further benefit seems to result. The goal of 200 minutes is an arbitrary one which several leading exercise instructors have chosen as a standard.

Your choice of a particular aerobic activity depends on your own desires and your recent level of fitness. The activity should be one that can be graded. That is, you should be able to easily and gradually increase the effort and the duration of the exercise.

What's the payoff for exercising regularly? The answer is marked improvement in the organs of your body and a demonstrable increase in physical well being. Among the changes are:

Brain — an improved sense of well being, less depression and anxiety.

Lungs — improved capacity to use oxygen and increased strength and endurance of breathing muscles.

Heart — stronger, more efficient heart muscle, more blood pumped with each heartbeat and slower resting pulse; collateral circulation expanded.

Muscles — increased strength, improved energy storage, better blood supply, improved capacity to take in and use oxygen and increased mobility and flexibility.

Bone — maintains it strength (density) and delays and, or, stops development of osteoporosis.

Tendons and ligaments — increased flexibility.

Body composition — less body fat and more lean body mass.

Hormones — lower blood sugar level, and lower adrenaline at rest (which decreases anxiety and muscle tension).

Coordination — improved reaction time and better balance.

Blood — increased oxygen carrying capacity, more efficient body cooling, increased blood volume, higher HDL (good) cholesterol level and lower triglyceride level.

Exercise should be fun. Often it doesn't seem so at first, but after your exercise habits are well developed, you will wonder how you ever got along without them.

Aerobic exercise refers to the kind of fast-paced activity that makes you huff and puff. It's good for you. It places demand on your body's cardiovascular apparatus and, over time, produces beneficial changes in your respiratory and circulatory systems.

There are three parameters under your control: frequency, distance or duration, and speed or intensity. Speed should always be considered last.

Frequency refers to how often you exercise.

Duration is the length of time devoted to each exercise session.

Intensity is a measurement of the level of your exertion during each workout.

Inactive women no matter what age should start with walking and then graduate to jogging, swimming and brisk walking as fits their individual desires. You always want to consult your doctor before starting an exercise program.

Develop exercise as a routine part of your day. For anybody, gentle activities performed daily are more beneficial and less likely to result in injury, particularly when getting started.

Many people will not want to exercise the 200 minutes a week. You can get most of the benefits with considerably less exercise. At 100 minutes per week you get almost 90 percent of the gain you get with 200 minutes. At 60 minutes per week you get 75 percent of the benefit you get with 200 minutes. Taking 100 minutes as a realistic goal for many women, consider that you are only taking about 20 minutes a day five days a week or about 15 minutes a day if you spread those 100 minutes over six days.

In the second part of this chapter, you'll meet Cherie and Jenine. Cherie is an out of shape woman who wants to prevent osteoporosis and her fitness instructor, Jenine takes her through the paces of gym exercises on athletic machines designed to stress the body and exercise the bones.

"This is totally boring." Cherie said to Jenine, who was orienting her to the health club. Jenine was showing Cheric how to use each piece of the equipment. "How can I make this enjoyable so I'll keep doing it?" questioned Cherie.

"Exercise can be a drag," answered Jenine. "Pedaling for an hour and not getting anywhere, pulling and pushing the padded handles of the machines can be an invitation to boredom unless you know how to make it enjoyable."

"First," she said, "don't try to find time for exercise, make a time for it like you do for a bath or shower. You wouldn't dream of going to work or for an outing without taking time to dress and straighten your hair. Start gently, and work up slowly," she continued. "So often in the past we saw clients for one or two weeks then they disappeared forever.

"Susan Powter says it accurately: 'Most fitness centers are too busy to focus on one individual, to make modifications in her program for sore knees, poor aerobic conditioning or address the fears than an overweight woman feels when she walks into an aerobic class filled with Barbie Doll-shaped figures.'

"We have been amiss in not giving proper attention and encouragement to new members," Jenine said to Cherie. "That's why I'm going to spend three hours with you over the next three days of orientation. I need to know your goals for the program and why you are here."

"I'm here to keep my bones hard and prevent osteoporosis," Cherie said. "Most of my aunts and my mother have had fractures and I don't want to have to deal with the problem later if I can prevent it. How can I go about it?"

"Preventing soft bones means keeping hard muscles," Jenine said. "Research shows that bone mass in the spine is proportional to the muscle strength of the back muscles, while hip bone strength is proportional to the strength of the quadriceps and hamstring muscles." (The front and back thigh muscles).

"You've had a good five minute warm up Cherie," Jenine said later. "Now lets do some stretches before we start challenging our muscles and ligaments. A muscle that's supple will be at low risk for tearing. Let's do the cat together. It'll loosen the soft tissues of your back, (muscles, ligaments, around the small joints and the fascia are like shrink wrap that holds the muscles in place).

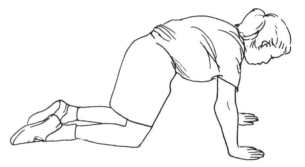

Illustration 42 – The Cat.

"Now for a few hamstring stretches; these are very important," said Jenine. "Do them standing up if you like it better than lying on the floor." (See page 72. You should feel the pull where you see the arrow.) "For your first day, we'll do these stretches, then use the machines."

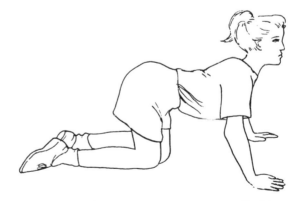

Illustration 43 – This position sometimes is called the camel as there are two humps.

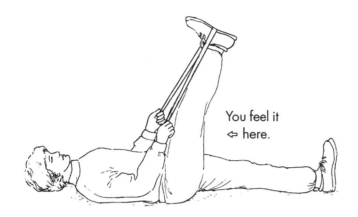

You feel it ⇦ here.

Illustration 44 – Hamstring Stretch lying down

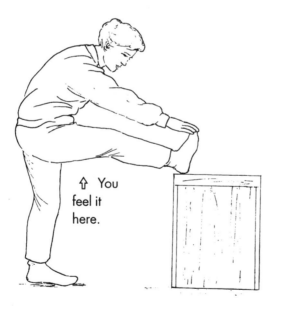

⇧ You feel it here.

Illustration 45 - Hamstring Stretch standing.

"There's nothing to this program," said Cherie. "It's easy and it won't take me all day."

"One of our local sports medicine doctors gave us an exercise prescription that is on the wall by the back machine," Jenine observed. "It reads, Rx: Make exercise part of your day. Start gently and work up. Make it fun, make it enjoyable. Pick your best time of day. Wear comfortable clothes. Reward your efforts frequently. Don't expect big results too soon. Persevere, you can do it."

"You mean exercise is supposed to be fun?" questioned Cherie.

"It's fun but it's also work when you use the machines. They hold you in a protective position while you work one set of muscles. The muscles work the bones," Jenine said.

"This ominous looking machine," Jenine continued, "is a back extensor strengthening unit or back machine. It's actually quite comfortable and will help you restore vigor to a stiff, weak back." We'll start with the lightest weight, 13 pounds."

"That feels too easy," Cherie said, so Jenine put on 3 plates or 39 pounds. As Jenine told Cherie, most women start at about 40 pounds on the Nautilus or Cybex back machine, but we want you to do it without straining and to be comfortable.

Thirty nine pounds was perfect and Cherie performed 10 repetitions with this weight. The last two were difficult.

"Right on," barked Jenine. "The last two pushes should challenge your muscles."

"Well, they did," Cherie said, wiping a few beads of perspiration from her forehead.

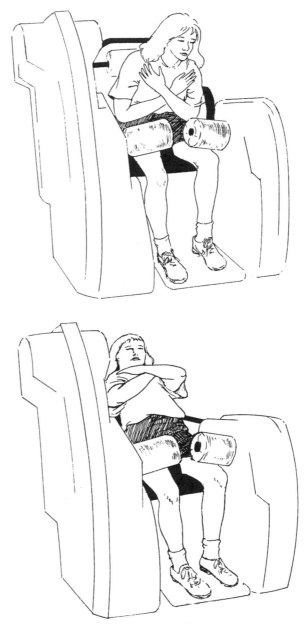

Illustrations 46 and 47 – Gym, Back Extension.

"Let's check out the quad and ham machines," Jenine suggested, taking her student over to the two machines that isolate the muscles of the front of thigh (quadriceps) and the back of the thigh (hamstrings). She pointed out how easy and smooth the movements are then encouraged Cherie to "Go ahead and do one set of 10 repetitions on each machine."

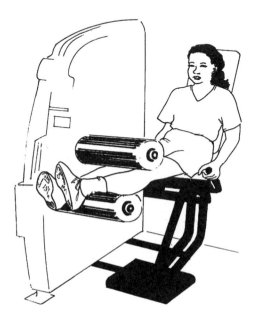

Illustration 48 – Gym, Hamstring.

This exercise strengthens the femur and muscles that cross the hip.

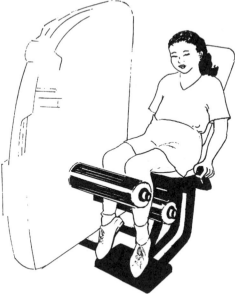

Illustration 49 – Gym, Hamstring.

Cherie gently worked the machines; the quad was the easiest while the hamstring was too difficult for her to move even one plate.

"Don't strain to do it," Jenine instructed. "We'll use some ankle weights for a week first to waken up those soft muscles."

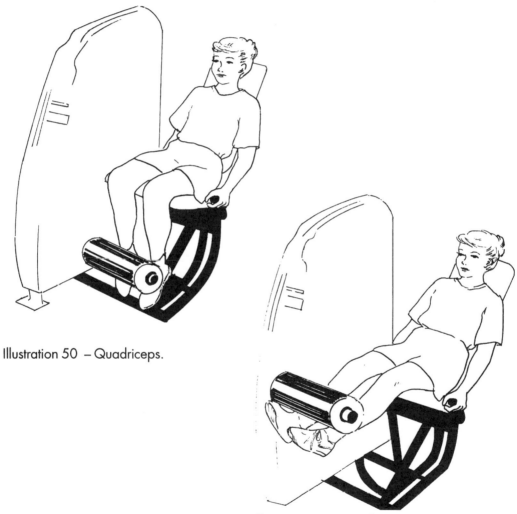

Illustration 50 – Quadriceps.

Illustration 51 – Quadriceps.

Both women walked to the free weight (non-machine) section and Jenine strapped a four pound weight on each of Cherie's ankles then told Cherie lie face down on an incline bench.

Cherie could pull the weights and felt relieved that she was able to do some exercises with her hamstring.

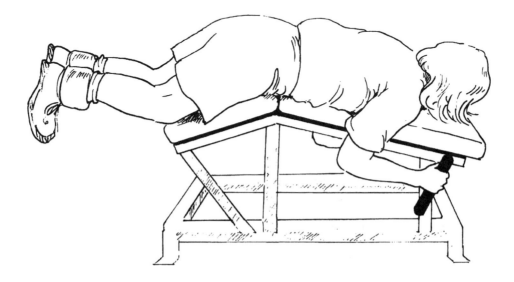

Illustration 52 – Incline Bench with Four Pound Ankle Weights for the Hamstrings.

Next, Jenine took Cherie to the treadmill where she showed her how to use it.

"This is a great exercise to prevent osteoporosis because of the weight bearing," she said. "Three miles per hour is the most efficient speed people walk but since you mentioned you haven't been doing much exercise, we'll start at two miles per hour with the machine flat."

It turned out that this speed was plenty for Cherie. After five minutes she felt a glow of perspiration, felt tired and stopped.

"Okay Cherie," Jenine said, "it's time for stretches, then you're finished."

"But Jenine, I thought we've already done stretches," Cherie said.

"Yes," answered Jenine, "we did stretches before strengthening to protect the muscles from injury. Now that you're all warmed up we'll stretch for flexibility." The stretches were easier this time and Jenine was careful to keep the stretches gentle.

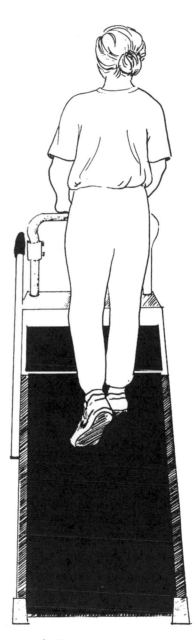

Illustration 53 – Treadmill.

"There's a spot on your exercise card to record your flexibility," Jenine said, pointing to the stretching box. She pointed out that on some days Cherie would be stiffer than others, but if she stuck with the program, she could actually observe her flexibility improve over a few weeks.

Cherie was a minus six when she started which means the tips of her fingers were six inches away from the stretching box. Her goal was to be at least zero, to be able to touch the box at the end of her toes.

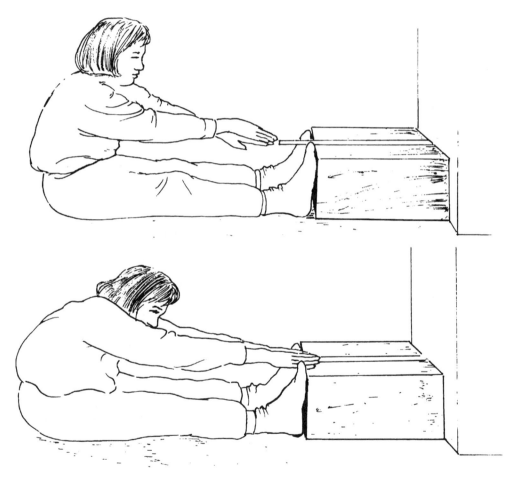

Illustrations 54 and 55 – Stretching Box, Inflexible and flexible.

"Out of shape hamstrings are the biggest challenge for clients, but you've shown that you can make them work for you,." Jenine remarked.

Cherie felt a glow in her face and she flushed slightly.

The exercises Jenine took Cherie through are the main ones that prevent osteoporosis. By the time any woman who is a beginner warms up, stretches, does three sets of 10 repetitions on the main machines, does aerobics and stretches again, she will have used up about an hour. If you want to use all the machines, go ahead. The ones we've described and illustrated in this chapter are the cornerstones of preventive exercise therapy. Three other exercises are included for overall strengthening. See page 80 to page 82. The rowing exercises strengthen the upper back. The pullover strengthens the abdomen and upper body while the lat pulldown strengthens the arms and shoulders.

The University of Florida Center for Exercise Science has published research that shows that stronger back extensor muscles equal stronger vertebrae in the back.

Stronger muscles around the wrist and arm mean stronger wrist bones and less likelihood of fracture. Stronger quadricep and hamstring muscles mean stronger hip bones, less fractures and more independence.

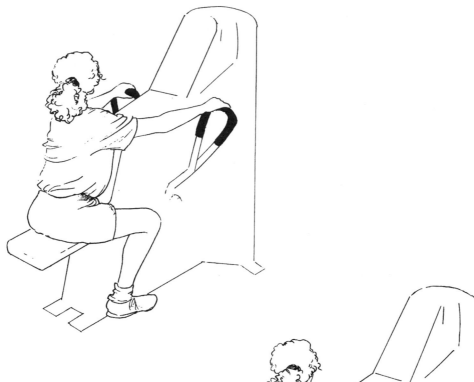

Illustrations 56 – Gym, Rowing.

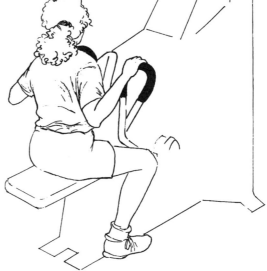

Illustrations 57 – Gym, Rowing.

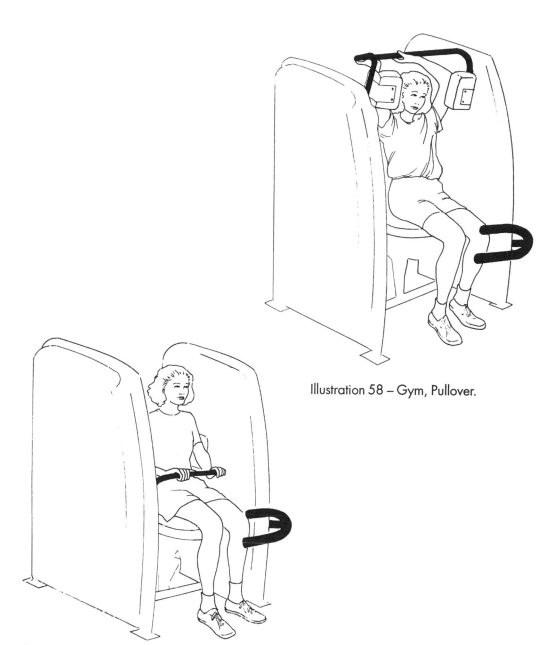

Illustration 58 – Gym, Pullover.

Illustration 59 – Gym, Pullover.

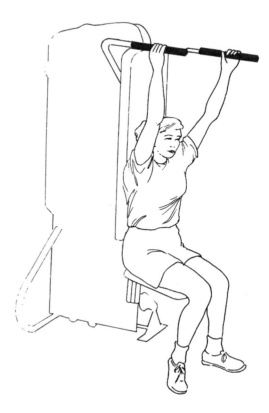

Illustration 60 – Gym, Lat Pulldown.

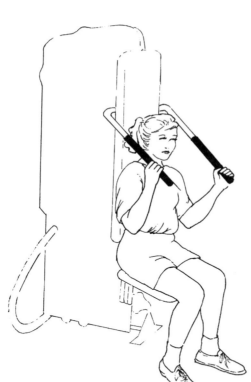

Illustration 61 – Gym, Lat Pulldown.

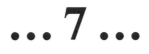

... 7 ...

Home Exercise Gym
To Prevent And Treat Osteoporosis

Brittle bones or body beautiful?

You'd like to participate in an exercise program but find it difficult to get to the gym with little ones at home and a job that demands much of your time. Take heart! There is an inexpensive home program to make your life easier. You can do the exercises alone or with family members or friends.

Does it sound impossible? Home gyms have become the rage in the last 10 years. What if you don't have $5,000 or more for fancy, chrome equipment? Easy, use the new home gym program you can make yourself for $10. All you need is an exercise band available at all sports stores and a piece of rope.

I wish you could see the marvelous growth changes bones undergo with exercise stress. Most of us, when we think of bones, visualize objects like the dried, bleached bones of the Texas Longhorns found in the desert country. But live bone is a growing, ever-changing organ under constant repair and change. When you exercise your muscles, you exercise your bones. How do bones work?

In growing children bone activity is greatest. A bone enzyme, alkaline phosphatase, is present in very high concentration during the growing years showing that there is high bone turnover and production.

After the formative years, bone activity decreases and only small amounts of alkaline phosphatase are found in the blood. Tests to determine the presence of alkaline phosphatase are usually performed on routine blood chemistry examinations when you have a physical. If you are fully-grown an elevated alkaline phosphatase reading indicates to your doctor that likely there are microfractures in your bones and new bone is forming. This is usually a sign of osteoporosis.

Bone responds to use and stress by laying down a frame of protein and then filling the protein frame with calcium. The process is like a house under construction. The 2 X 4 frame is the protein and the walls are the calcium filling in the space in and around the 2 X 4 frame to add strength to the bone.

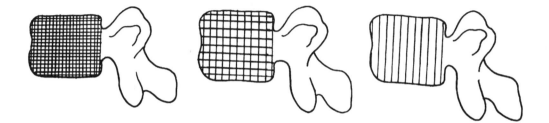

Illustrations 85, 86 and 87 – The Amount of New Bone Formation Dwindles.

Just as a house deteriorates over time unless it is kept up with continued maintenance, bones deteriorate without regular stress applied to them. With double-income families more common each year and after hours devoted to laundry, cooking and cleaning, exercise has taken a back seat to work and home activities.

As I wrote in an earlier chapter, in order for a woman to stay healthy she must exercise, and that requires making exercise not a duty, but an integral part of a living program.

A program at home starts with exercise activities that are designed to stretch and strengthen particular parts of the body. Remember, while you are strengthening muscles, you are stressing bones — making them stronger, healthier and more resistant to disease.

We'll show each of the strengthening activities recommended at the beginning and at the finish.

Always start with a warm up. The extra blood created in a warm up loosens muscles and opens tiny capillaries which supply nutrients and help prevent injury. Walk around the house for five minutes or go up and down the stairs a few times. Use a bike or a ski machine for a few minutes. Now you are ready.

Stretching before strengthening helps prevent pulls and strains of the muscles. A warm, flexible muscle is less prone to tearing or spasming. See the stretches on pages 85 to 90.

For the shoulder stretch, use a rope or sport band. Stand, hold ends of the rope or band and slowly extend arms overhead. For comfort, wrap bands around knuckles and fingers. Slowly bring arms down and behind the head, keeping them wide for resistance. Bring arms up slowly and repeat. Start with the band in front of the shoulders then move upward and over the shoulders toward the back.

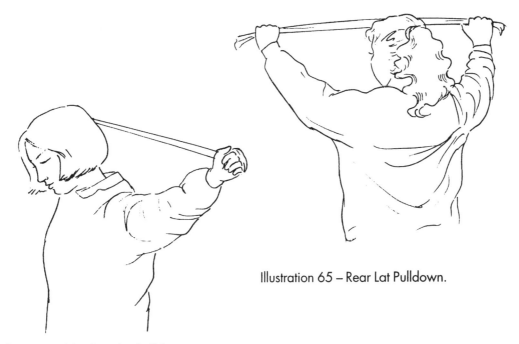

Illustration 65 – Rear Lat Pulldown.

Illustration 66 – Rear Lat Pulldown.

Next, try the yoga twist for paraspinal and abdominal muscles. Seated, extend the right leg and cross the left over it, holding the left knee back with the right arm, twisting around with the head and upper body and looking left. Hold for at least 15 seconds, release and switch sides.

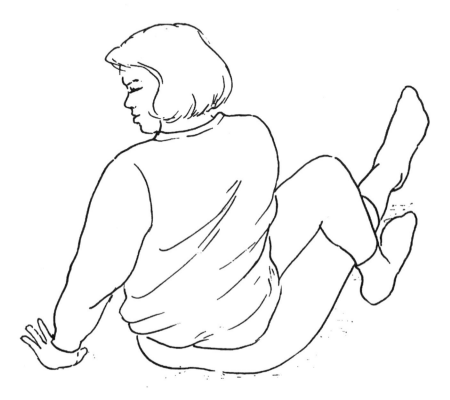

Illustration 67 – Yoga Twist.

The cat can teach you about stretching. This movement stretches the paraspinal muscles and the lower back and abdomen. On hands and knees, head level to spine, round your back by pulling the abdominal muscles toward the ceiling, then reverse the neutral position: imagine a cat stretching. Repeat three times. See page 71.

The sphinx was developed to help create supple abdominal and back muscles. Lie on your stomach with your elbows under your shoulders. Slowly press up keeping the stomach muscles firm without straining your back. Come up to forearms, hold for 10 seconds, release down. Repeat three times.

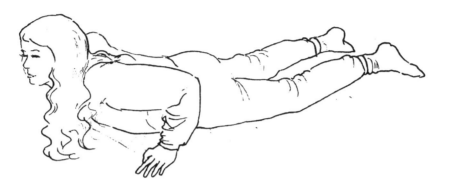

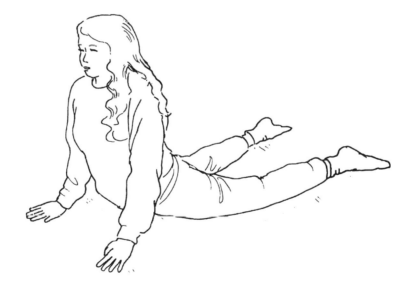

Illustrations 68 and 69 – Sphinx.

Hip flexors exercises help to prevent falls and to keep the hip flexors and thighs supple. This exercise will improve balance and coordination. Lie on your back on a pad or floor. Bring your right knee into your chest. Hold for at least 15 seconds, breathing deeply. Repeat with the left leg.

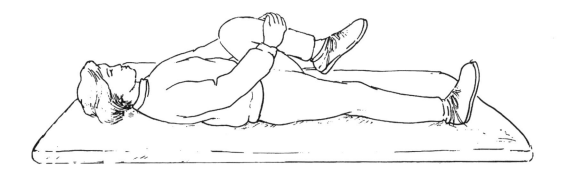

Illustration 70 – Hip Flexion.

For the abdominal crunch, lie on your back with your knees bent and your feet flat on the floor. Reach up with your hands until your shoulder blades are off the floor and feel the contracting abdominal muscles tighten as they push your low back into the floor. Release slightly and repeat the contraction in a pulsing action, 10 to 15 times. Add a twist to each side for 10 to 15 repetitions.

Pull straight
forward.

Pull to the
right side.

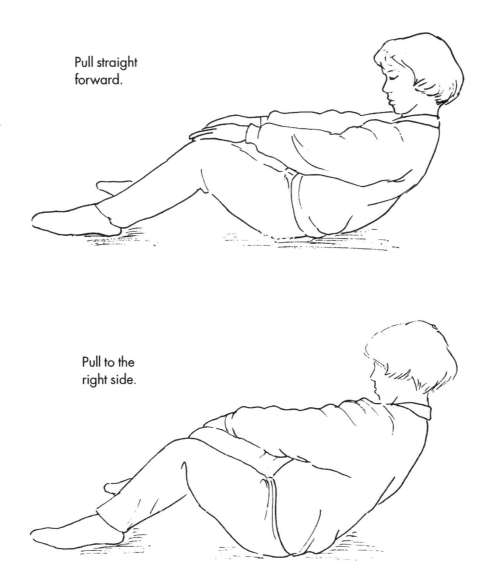

Illustrations 71 and 72 – Abdominal Crunch.

Biceps and triceps. Since fractures of the wrist are common, you'll want to keep these bones hard. Sitting in a chair, put your Theraband under your feet with your arms parallel to your thighs. Now pull the band up using your bicep muscles. Do three sets of ten repetitions for all exercises for a total of 30 repetitions. It may be easier to alternate the biceps and triceps.

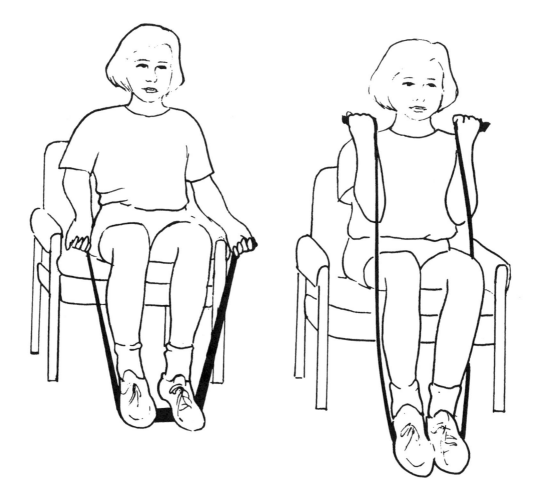

Illustrations 73 and 74 – Biceps.

For the triceps, sit in a chair with the band around the back of your chair. You'll need about five feet of the band for these exercises. Now extend or straighten your elbows and feel the pull on the back of your upper arms.

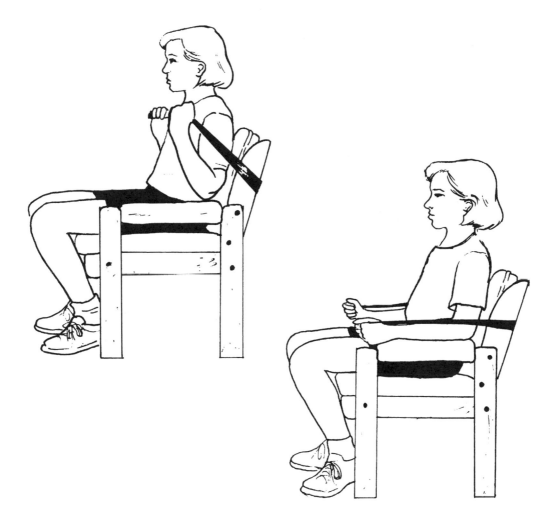

Illustrations 75 and 76 – Triceps.

To strengthen the back muscles, sit in a comfortable chair or on the couch and push backward with your body into the couch. For the side abdominal and back muscles, do a slight twist during the backward push. Do three sets of 10 repetitions.

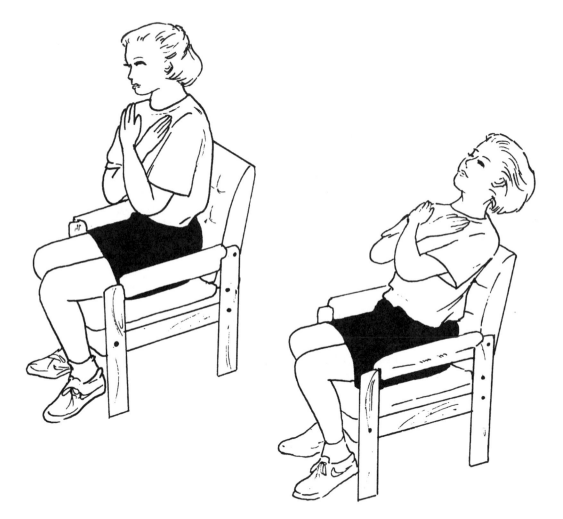

Illustrations 77 and 78 – Back Strengthening.

Abdominal muscles are often neglected, and of course the fat around your middle is really due to months and years of poor eating habits and inadequate exercise. How many fat marathon runners do you see? Let's work on the abdomen and wake it up.

Sit in your exercise chair and wrap a band around your chair as you did for the triceps but instead of holding the band at your sides, cross your arms in front of you. Now lean forward and push against the force of the band.

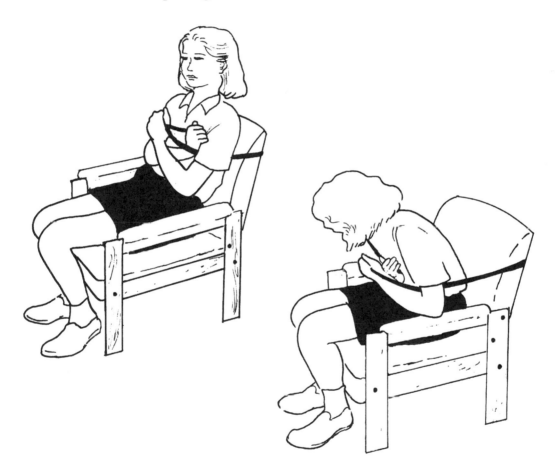

Illustrations 79 and 80 – Abdominal Muscles.

Row, row, row your back. Sit on the floor in the rowing position with your knees slightly bent to keep the strain off the lower back nerves. Gently pull or rock backward against the sport band. If it feels too easy, shorten the sport band. If it is too difficult, then use a longer piece of sport band.

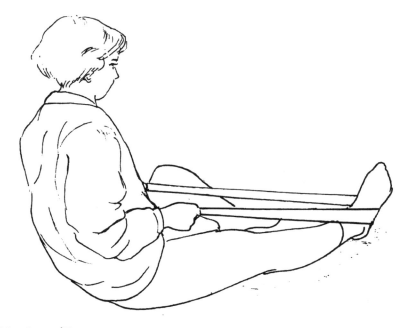

Illustration 81 – Seated Row.

For leg strengthening, use the sport band tied and wrapped around a sturdy chair leg for resistance. For the quadricep muscle on the front of the thigh, set up the band as you see in Illustrations 82 and 83 Stretch and hold for 10 seconds while resisting with the other leg.

In the past, it was thought that the quadricep muscle should be much stronger than the hamstring muscle on the back of the thigh, but now studies show the two of them should be more equal in strength. I can't guarantee you'll look like a cover girl after doing these exercises, but you will feel invigorated and will experience a warm flush as fresh oxygen-rich blood is delivered to the muscles. These exercises can even be performed while watching television if you desire.

This home exercise program is inexpensive, easy to use and invigorating to stale muscles. Exercising in the comfort of your home adds a degree of flexibility and saves the driving and dressing time involved in athletic club programs. Whether you chose exercise at home or prefer working out at a gym with the social contacts such an atmosphere provides, the important rule to remember is constancy. Make your exercises as important to your life as brushing your teeth or shampooing your hair. In a few weeks you'll start to feel firmer and those little rings of fat will start to shrink making way for strong muscles to keep your bones hard.

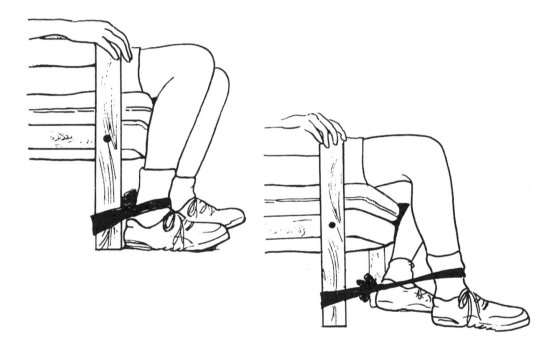

Illustrations 82 and 83 – Quadriceps strengthening.

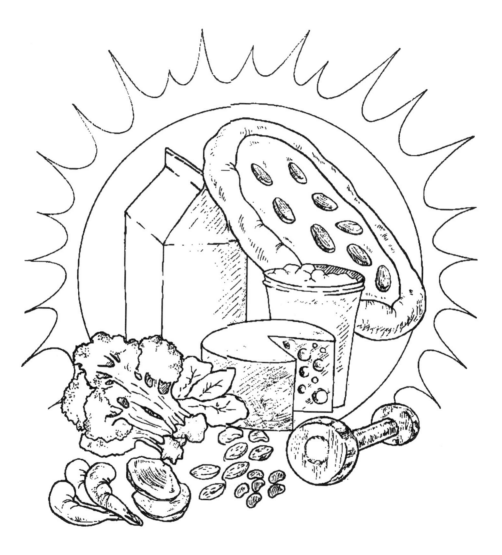

Illustration 84 – Foods High in Calcium and in Micronutrients.

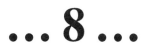

... 8 ...

Micronutrients and
Their Role in Keeping Bones Hard

What can you do to build and maintain dense bones other than by increasing your intake of calcium and doing more exercises? Several nutritional maneuvers can help toughen up your bones and add to their density. A proper, balanced diet can make us all healthier in a general sense, but we need to be more specific if we're dealing with osteoporosis.

Normally, the body contains about three pounds of calcium. Our goal is to keep that calcium in the body, especially in the bones. Phosphorus is a key element in retention of calcium in the bones. Your body needs phosphorus to utilize calcium efficiently. Three fourths of the phosphorus is in the bones, the remaining amount is in the other soft tissues, especially the nerves and skin. Phosphorus and calcium are inversely related in the blood. As the phosphorus level increases, the calcium level decreases.

In the digestive tract, excess phosphorus combines with calcium and they form calcium phosphate which the body cannot absorb, so the calcium goes to waste. Your body's requirements after 40 years of age indicate a need for more calcium and less phosphorus. Following is a list of foods high in phosphorus and they should be eaten sparingly: red meat, carbonated soft-drinks, beef liver, bologna, hot dogs and ham. The more time that lapses between eating these foods and your intake of calcium-rich foods, the better your chance of absorbing the calcium you ingest. There is no shortage of phosphorus in the average diet so you do not need to supplement yours with phosphorus.

The problem: medical research is often years ahead of the medical textbooks your health care provider reads. By the time your physician reads information in a medical book, the research usually is five to six years old. Research in the field of osteoporosis continues to develop new information, but there is a lag between discovery and application. Journals are published monthly that contain short articles to summarize the work of researchers and frequently much of the material is shortened or omitted. But I've included in this book current research information to keep you abreast of the "natural" way to treat osteoporosis.

Our Western diet, filled with refined foods, combines with environmental pollution and with decreased appetite and slower intestinal absorption in the elderly to produce *nutritional osteoporosis.* To prevent this disease, I recommend adding known micronutrients to the diet, and avoiding those known dietary causes of osteoporosis which I've already discussed, such as alcohol and caffeine. Hippocrates said: "Let your food be your medicine and let your medicine be your food." Nutritional medicine involves reducing junk food in your diet while increasing fruits, vegetables and whole grains. This may not be enough as we age.

Sugar, alcohol, caffeine and salt are all associated with osteoporosis, and when they are ingested more than sparingly they add to nutritional deficits. As they are increased in the diet — and since they contain no significant vitamins or minerals — the result to the body is less Vitamin C, magnesium, zinc and other important nutrients. By eating only two candy bars, you can cause an increase in calcium excretion which helps to soften the bones. The occasional candy bar does not cause problems, but there is a serious potential problem with the daily intake of hundreds of extra calories of refined sugar.

Dr. John Yudkin, an English physician, who studied the effect of sucrose (table sugar) on osteoporosis, stated that a high sucrose intake raises our body's production of cortisol (the body's natural cortisone). Over the years this can result in softer bones in the same way that taking prescription cortisone in low doses can cause loss of calcium from the bones.

The big discovery in nutritional science is the role "K" plays in osteoporosis. To understand its important function in bone building, you need to know that Vitamin K is as important for your bones as calcium. Vitamin K is needed for blood clotting and is called the *Koagulation* vitamin. When the body tissues are injured, clotting factors in the blood go to the injury site and are acted upon by Vitamin K to produce a clot and slow and stop the bleeding.

Vitamin K also is present in green, leafy vegetables, and any reasonably healthy diet contains some Vitamin K. Bowel bacteria also produce Vitamin K, so very few of us have bleeding disorders. However antibiotics can cause bleeding and bone loss if used for any length of time because they kill normal bacterial that produce Vitamin K. Newer antibiotics are so powerful that they have become capable of nearly sterilizing the gut with resulting severe bleeding problems. Preoccupation with bleeding problems caused physicians to overlook as inconsequential the effect of Vitamin K on the bones. As a result, the osteoporotic effects of loss of Vitamin K were not determined until years later.

Now we know how important Vitamin K is for the production of osteocalcin, a protein found in large quantities in the bone. I mentioned earlier that the protein framework of the bones is similar to 2 x 4s in the walls of a house. The protein that makes the framework is osteocalcin, on which crystals of minerals form to make the bones hard. Vitamin K causes the protein osteocalcin to become "sticky" which helps calcium ions become attracted and attached to it. The movement of calcium to the bone mineral matrix is an important step in building hard bones and in bone repair after microfractures that occur with our activities of daily living. Administering Vitamin K can diminish the calcium loss in the urine by up to 50 percent. A recent study from the Netherlands measured the capacity of osteocalcin to bind calcium crystal in the bone. Postmenopausal women whose calcium level dropped to one half of normal values recovered to normal status when their diets were supplemented with Vitamin K. Also, the study pointed out that premenopausal women usually had normal levels of Vitamin K.

As a result of antibiotic potency, it is recommended that you take Vitamin K after you have taken a prescription of antibiotics. If you are one of the unlucky people to be taking daily antibiotics for acne or other chronic infection, then be absolutely sure to take extra Vitamin K. See the recommendations for dosage at the end of this chapter.

Since aging causes a decrease in food intake and absorption of food from the intestine, if you are over 50 years of age, then you should start taking a supplement with Vitamin K and the other vitamins and minerals recommended in this chapter. If at present you are taking medicine to prevent blood clotting, like coumadin or warfarin, then talk to your doctor before taking any Vitamin K because it may interfere with your prescription.

What other trace minerals are important to bone health?

Manganese is a trace mineral that is needed for bone repair. It is useful in the production of mucopolysaccharides from which the protein-like molecules of bone are made. If your manganese level is low, then your formation of mucopolysaccharides will be decreased and the process of bone remodeling and bone repair will be impaired and delayed.

Food processing techniques cause loss of manganese, so if you eat processed foods regularly, then supplement them with manganese. Manganese occurs naturally in rice polish or the skin (bran) of brown rice. Most Westerners do not eat large amounts of rice and if they do they often use rice without polish or rice whose skin has been removed. If you eat white rice, polished rice is best.

Often magnesium and manganese are confused as they sound somewhat alike, but it is imperative to keep them separated in your mind so you don't overdose on manganese. Overdosing on manganese can produce psychiatric symptoms such as hallucinations, anxiety and memory changes. Follow the recommendations at the end of this chapter when choosing your vitamins and minerals. The rule for manganese is that if a small amount is useful, a larger amount is toxic.

Magnesium is the mineral that balances calcium in the body. It is needed for all energy-producing reactions in the body. Any type of stress, whether physical or emotional, can release magnesium into the blood stream and allow it to be excreted by the kidney. The Recommended Daily Allowance is 350 mg. per day, but most people consume one third less than this. Magnesium is depleted by alcohol, diuretics used for treating edema, and by digoxin, a pill used to control heart rate and the strength of heart contractions. Fifty percent of the body's magnesium is found in the bone.

Osteoporosis researchers Cohen and Kitzes performed magnesium challenge tests and those patients who retained 90 percent of the intravenous dose were thought to be low in magnesium. When magnesium is low, the quality of the magnesium crystals are less than optimal, which can result in abnormal mineralization of the bones. Usually, calcium is supplemented in a two to one ratio with magnesium. If you take in 1200 mg. of calcium, you should take in 600 mg. of magnesium. There is no single nutrient that functions alone in the body and by paying attention to each nutrient as part of the whole, you can make your food your medicine.

Another physician, Guy Abraham, M. D., supplemented the diets of women with 500 mg. of calcium citrate and 600 mg. of magnesium oxide for nine months and they showed an increase in bone mass of 11 percent versus a loss of about one percent in the untreated group.

However, the patients were also exercising, eating a healthy diet, and avoiding alcohol, caffeine, tobacco and extra salt and sugar. There is no one single treatment that acts to prevent osteoporosis or that treats it when it is present, but the combinations described can be a life saver to those afflicted with this problem.

Magnesium occurs in high concentrations in whole grains, nuts, seeds, green vegetables and meat. The RDA is 350 mg. per day. Take at least this dosage to keep your bones hard. If you take too much magnesium it will cause diarrhea. When vitamins and minerals are taken in higher than recommended dosages, they have side effects the same as drugs. Magnesium also builds up in the blood if you have kidney damage or poor kidney function. If you do have kidney problems, consult your physician before taking extra magnesium.

Zinc is another trace mineral needed by the body in small amounts. Low zinc levels are often associated with recurrent infections, growth retardation, including bone-growth retardation, and slowed wound healing. Zinc enhances the activity of Vitamin D in bones and in the formation of osteoblasts that build bone. Since the jaw bone seems to be affected early in osteoporosis (osteoporosis of the mouth), and zinc levels are often low in osteoporosis, the idea has developed that zinc can help promote and maintain healthier, harder bones, including the jaw bone. A little zinc is helpful, but high doses can cause hemolytic anemia, a breakdown of red blood cells. Keep zinc levels at or below 50 mg. daily.

The trace mineral boron acts in an unusual and helpful way when treating osteoporosis. In one research study, postmenopausal women were maintained on a low boron diet for four months by avoiding fruits, vegetables and nuts. Next, they were supplemented with three mg. of boron daily and their urinary excretion of calcium dropped by 40 percent. Boron assists in the conversion of Vitamin D to its active form, 1,25-Hydroxy Vitamin D. If you eat fruits, vegetables and nuts daily, you are probably getting enough boron. If you don't eat them regularly, then supplement with one mg. of boron per day.

Boron is a trace mineral and you only need a small amount of it. While the toxic dose is over 100 times the recommended dose of one mg., just remember, a little goes a long way. Don't overdose yourself.

Why do people become deficient in boron if it is so easy to consume fruits, vegetables and nuts daily? For one thing, nuts have developed a bad press because they are high in fat and fat in our environment is not acceptable, so women avoid them. Fruits and vegetables are consumed in quantity during the summer months, but in the winter the cost of fruits increase and some people on fixed incomes must be very cautious when spending money on fruit.

How does Vitamin C fit in the scheme of osteoporosis? Deficiency of Vitamin C can cause scurvy, a disease in which the connective tissue of the body weakens and breaks down. In the bones, Vitamin C causes stronger cross links in the protein framework. In general, 500 mg. to 1,000 mg. of Vitamin C per day will help keep bones hard, but if you have kidney problems, consult your physician before taking any supplement.

Bone and Its Battle Against Hydrogen

"Life is a struggle, not against sin, not against the money power, not against malicious animal magnetism, but against hydrogen ions." These words, written about the meaning of life and death by H. L. Mencken, refer to the damage that acid can cause to our skeletons.

Buffering by bone helps neutralize the long-term acid loading from our diet. Total acid excretion is lower than total acid production resulting in a positive acid balance. Additional acid in the body produces increased activity by osteoclasts, the cells that break down bone.

Bone has a large reservoir of alkaline salts and sodium and potassium ions that are available to buffer the hydrogen ions in acid. The total carbonate reservoir of bone can buffer retained acid, but the trade off is the loss of mineral from bone. Sebastian researched the effect of the Western diet on osteoporosis and found that when patients were given potassium bicarbonate, the acid production was neutralized, the calcium excretion decreased and the level of osteocalcin, or bone protein, increased. Research shows that the preserved bones of people of previous generations had more density at older ages than do the bones of the aging contemporary Westerner. This seems to suggest that our ancestors, who consumed less meat and more vegetables than we do now, had healthier bones. Processed food and environmental contaminants seem to be responsible for an increasing acid or hydrogen overload on our systems. It was popular, part of our national consciousness, in the 1950s to feed ourselves on a diet of meat and potatoes. Meat protein was ideal and a goal to achieve to prove that you were successful.

Now we know that the meat protein ingested over the years produced byproducts that were laden with hydrogen or weak acids. The most powerful buffering system in the body is the calcium which can be leached from the bones to help neutralize the acids. Over decades, the calcium leaching has caused less dense bones. Vegetarians have harder bones than meat eaters.

A newer source of hydrogen challenge to the bones may threaten you in the form of acid rain. I am sure you may be tired of hearing about acid rain and how it damages plants, trees and small animals in the environment, but some research experts are suggesting that acid rain can slowly suck the calcium out of your bones.

Acid rain is produced from hydrogen in the environment which combines with sulfur and oxygen to produce weak sulfuric acid. It also combines with nitrogen and oxygen to form nitric acid and it combines with carbon dioxide and oxygen to produce carbonic acid. Usually rainwater is slightly acidic with a pH of 5.6 or so. Neutral is a pH of 7.0. When the pH or amount of acid drops below 5.6 we have acid rain. Much of the acid rain is caused by burning coal in the environment to produce energy.

Cities attempt to keep their water supplies balanced and away from the acid side, but often the "natural" water sources such as a home well and country water sources can become acidic. If you have any doubts about the acidity of your own water, the city will test your water for you.

We can't possibly avoid all of the hydrogen or acid in the environment, but by applying common sense we can make decisions that will maintain healthy bodies and strong bones to support us through many decades of life. We can't change our past, but with a little nutritional maneuvering we can change our future.

Our Recommended Daily Dosages for Nutrient Supplementation Are:

Calcium	1,000 mg. – 1,500 mg.
Magnesium	500 mg. – 600 mg.
Zinc	25 mg. – 50 mg.
Manganese	5 mg. – 10 mg.
Vitamin K	250 mcg. – 500 mcg. (micrograms, not milligrams)
Vitamin C	500 mg. – 1,000 mg.
Vitamin D	400 units
Boron	1 mg.

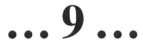

...9...

Preventing Osteoporosis:
Starting In The Teens

Twelve to twenty, those were the years. Football games and parties, dances and cars, the first taste of independence. The Barbie Doll ethic.

Ten pounds of excess weight to a sixteen-year-old may affect her self image the same way fifty extra pounds affects yours. At any one time, 80 percent of teenage girls are on a diet. Peer pressure is at its apex. How do you fill growing bones with calcium when your daughter is trying to melt into a pair of size five jeans? You know she isn't going to eat much, so what can you do?

Shop with prevention in mind. Keep low-fat, high- calcium foods on hand. Look for high-calcium foods like calcium-enriched orange juice, cereals, desserts, and green, leafy vegetables for salads. Most bone density is formed in these years so it's important to keep those bones stimulated. How?

If your daughter is thin because she avoids fats and exercises daily, she's at lower risk for later fractures. If she's thin because she starves herself through frequent dieting or she throws up, she's in trouble.

Encourage your daughter to participate in sports. The days of the boys playing and the girls watching are vanishing. Take advantage of school programs. Lifelong fitness classes have started in many schools to introduce students to individual sports like tennis, golf, swimming, hiking, bicycling, archery, body building and dancing. These activities can be continued throughout life after soccer and basketball teams have long since vanished.

Encourage all sports, team and individual. Rent a boat and take your daughter water skiing. Take a hike for an adventure, invite one of her friends. Sign her up for lessons early before she has preconceived ideas about what is feminine and what is not. If your daughter has lessons early, she'll perform better in relation to her friends and will feel good about participating.

Rent a sailboat and go sailing, the process of hiking-out or hanging over the side of the boat as a counterbalance will strengthen back and abdominal muscles. Kayak or canoe a local river to enjoy the scenery.

The Five Percent Rule

We spend 95 percent of our time indoors. By decreasing that time to 90 percent, you can decrease your daughter's chance of suffering from powdery bones. Get out, get active, get a life. Don't send your daughter, take her. The families that play together stay together.

Put up a basketball hoop and keep a jump rope around. Play catch with a softball. For the colder months with an "r" in their names, keep a Nordic Track or other exercise machine in the television room. If it is in the way and it's quiet, it'll be used more often. Show your daughter by example, don't tell her what to do. She'll love you for it.

... 10 ...

The Other Osteoporosis

Medical advances have made it possible to live into the nineties and we see weekly articles about centenarians celebrating their birthdays surrounded by friends and relatives. It is ironic that while people may now live longer, they may not live better since the skeleton decays and the rejuvenation of the bones seems beyond our reach.

These bones may last a "lifetime" but there is no guarantee about quality bone mass as the frail elderly suffer from skeletal debility.

Both sexes begin losing bone mass at about age 35 and lose about 1 percent each year thereafter. Women lose 3 percent for each of the next ten years following the menopause so without treatment, by age 60, a woman has lost 45 percent of her bone mass and a man has lost 25 percent. By age 80 a woman has lost 65 percent of her bone mass and a man has lost 45 percent. By age 100, women have lost 85 percent of her bone mass and men have lost 65 percent.

Unless these elderly individuals have continued to exercise and make healthy life choices, they will suffer from skeletal incompetence leading to fractures from minor traumas like sneezing. You've watched very old men and women walk with tiny steps and with a wide stance to prevent falling, the ultimate fear of the elderly.

When they fall it is like watching a building collapse with the same result. Their skeletons have failed them. The Humpty-Dumpty syndrome; all the kings horses and all the kings men can't put this person together again.

What has happened to these individuals who were full of zest for life but now sit in the rocker or recliner "to be safe." The move to the recliner has taken the risk out of life but has often taken the life out of life. They watch movies and identify with characters that can live their lives for them.

What is happening that we can't enjoy the time of our life when we have children, grandchildren and great grandchildren? Life should offer more than a chance to sit on the sofa and slowly lose our vitality as our bones dissolve from under us.

Senile osteoporosis; even the name suggests the end of life. Who suffers from this? Can you prevent it? The answer is "Yes," if you understand how the bones work.

Osteoporosis is a problem with defective remodeling units. Look at the side picture of the healthy vertebra shown on page 109 and notice the force lines running vertically and horizontally. The tiny squares between the lines are about the size of a remodeling unit (RMU). Each of these squares or remodeling units is constantly developing microfractures and each one is in a state of healing or remodeling. The amount of new bone formation dwindles as we age, especially with inactivity. It normally takes three to four months for a remodeling unit to break down the old bone and form new bone and lay down calcium crystals along the protein framework. With senile osteoporosis, the remodeling unit takes from two to four years to complete its work, eight to twelve times as long as expected. This absolutely does not need to occur, so why does it? Why not delay the development of soft, incompetent bones until past the time when you no longer need them.

Osteoporosis can't be delayed forever but it can be delayed until you have lived your life to the fullest and accomplished your goals. Eventually, we must all die of something, but most of us would choose to live life like an alkaline battery with nearly full power until the light goes out, versus the regular battery that gets weaker and dimmer and slowly extinguishes.

This chapter, addressed to older readers, includes some technical information, but it is mainly centered on the theme that it is perfectly possible for you to develop "Bone Power" even at advanced ages. "How can that be?" you ask. The answer lies in a definition of what happens to aging bones. In summary, elderly inactivity plus chronic calcium deficiency, combined with inadequate amounts of estrogen or testos-

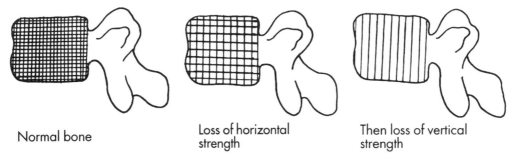

| Normal bone | Loss of horizontal strength | Then loss of vertical strength |

Illustrations 62, 63 and 64 – Healthy Bone And Bone Deterioration.

terone and compounded by decreased Vitamin D activity and increased parathyroid hormone production, occur at a time when our heredity catches up with us. You'll need to read the definition again for the complete impact to come through. Summarizing the aging process of the bones sounds like medical hocus pocus, but in the next few pages I'll discuss each part of it so you can enjoy "Bone Power" instead of "bone powder".

All right. First, you have to understand about abnormal bone physiology. Quality bones cannot be produced or maintained unless there is an adequate supply of building materials such as calcium and protein. Bone turnover is determined by how many bone modeling units are being formed versus how many are being uncoupled. Earlier, I mentioned that osteoblasts build bone while osteoclasts crush or destroy bone. We need to maintain an equilibrium between the activities of these two cell groups.

I mentioned estrogen deficiency as a cause of soft bones. Estrogen prevents reabsorption of bone by parathyroid hormone. In its absence, more parathyroid hormone softens the bones. Another irony is that low doses of parathyroid hormone harden bones while high doses soften bone.

As we age, we tend to take in less Vitamin D. This important vitamin is added to commercial milk supplies in North America and Sweden and can also be made by your skin when it is exposed to the sun for 20 minutes, with the sun's rays acting on the oil in the skin. Many people, concerned about sunshine-induced skin cancer do not venture into the sun without skin covering of one type or another. As a result, unless you live in a semi-tropical area, you are not likely to have sun exposure most of the year. Now, here's what's important: low levels of Vitamin D will decrease your absorption of calcium. The blood levels of calcium will drop and the bones will be called on to donate more stored calcium to maintain blood levels.

As we age, our kidney functions slowly deteriorate resulting in less absorption of calcium and more absorption of phosphorus. As the phosphorus increases, the serum calcium decreases and more calcium is drawn out of the bones. In addition, high phosphorus intake, which comes from eating meat as a food source, causes this same imbalance and loss of calcium. The rate of bone loss is greater in omnivores than in vegetarians who avoid meat which is the main source of phosphorus. It should be obvious by now that loss of calcium is critical to healthy bones. The loss has to be replaced through an osteoporosis medical management plan. One part of that plan is calcitonin, a thyroid hormone that keeps bones hard. Calcitonin levels decrease with age and along with them come dwindling bone mass. Sex hormones help maintain higher levels of calcitonin but these hormones also decrease with age. Calcitonin is available in injectable form and in some areas it can be purchased as a nasal spray or as rectal suppositories to be used three times per week at a dose of 100-200 units. Calcitonin rehardens softening bones. It also can increase bone density up to 8 percent in twelve months. In injectable form, at least 100 units of salmon calcitonin are required every other day to harden bones. Usually, within a year your body will build antibodies to salmon calcitonin so it is usually only effective the first time it is used.

Why can a bone suddenly give out with minimal trauma? As you study the side view of the vertebrae and hip bones and the strength lines, note the decrease in lines of force that maintain bone integrity. This happens with aging. A reduction of bone density to one third normal causes a loss of one-ninth of bone strength. A decrease of density to one half normal results in a loss of one fourth of bone strength. By age 80 in both sexes the bones are delicate and mere shells of their former selves. Osteoporosis can't be avoided forever, but it can be postponed until late in life with specific physical and medical maneuvers.

Reductions in bone mass are not always painful. Sometimes the vertebrae slowly crush into themselves as frequent microfractures occur. These silent fractures may be painless. However, if there is a sudden fracture as a vertebra crushes into itself, there is excruciating pain.

In the elderly age group, exercise is just as important as a deterrent to osteo-porosis as it is to younger persons. But, how much exercise is enough for persons in their advanced years? We all are aware that we should exercise but for most folks who want to get away with minimums, here are recommended levels of physical activity. It is crucial to maintain good posture, cardiorespiratory fitness and endurance by including low-impact aerobics, walking, and stationary exercise bicycling or active bicycling. Stretching and extension or backward bending exercises are helpful to maintain mobility. Well-planned exercise programs can improve bone mass on densitometer studies.

Hip bone density is higher in athletes and the density is related to the intensity of exercise. Aerobic dance is more successful than a walking program. In a 140-pound individual, walking will generate up to 700 pounds of force with the impact of the foot on the ground. Aerobic dance may increase its force up to two or three times. The amount of bone density is related to the amount of stress or work you put on the skeleton.

Cavanaugh and associates in the journal BONE in 1988 showed that brisk walking for 15-40 minutes *three times* a week for 42 weeks failed to prevent bone loss of the skeleton in early post menopausal women. More intense exercise does have a beneficial effect on bone mass. Thirty minutes of exercise *daily* consisting of walking, jogging, or dancing or an exercise program of ten to fifteen minutes of strengthening isometrically (without movement), or with weights will definitely improve bone density. One hour of *aerobic* exercise per day three times per week will prevent bone loss.

Aerobic means exercising at 80 percent of your maximum heart rate for one hour. To determine your maximum heart rate, subtract your age from 220. Exercise has been shown to increase bone density by 2 percent per year over a two year period. If exercise is stopped, the bones once again begin to soften.

In individuals taking Biphosphonates for a year, they increased bone density by 4.5 percent. The following years the bones did not increase in density but did not lose density.

Vitamin D3 at a dose of 800 units per day, plus 1000mg of calcium daily given to 84-year-old nursing home residents in France decreased hip fractures by 50 percent. No benefit was shown by taking only 400 units of Vitamin D3.

It appears that finally at a time in our lives when we have more time to ourselves we need to spend one hour daily exercising. But when you measure the benefits — a more vigorous lifestyle without the fear of powdery bones that may break if you sneeze too hard — that hour is a small price to pay. You don't need to go to a health club. Purchase a few free weights such as dumbbells or wear wrist weights while exercising to increase the stress on your bones. In the older age group it takes extra vigilance and exercise determination to keep osteoporosis at bay. One hour a day.

We have discussed estrogen and its effect on the bones and mentioned testosterone-estrogen preparations. Studies have shown that estrogen increases bone density by 4.5 percent per year for a two year period, while untreated individuals lost another three percent of bone mass. This means that with two years of estrogen therapy, the bones are 12 percent harder than non-treated individuals. (4.5 + 4.5 = 9 percent) this calculates to be nine percent above pretreatment levels versus a three percent loss in untreated individuals. This hormonal therapy can be effective even when introduced up to 35 years after menopause.

Another treatment that has been successful is the use of anabolic steroids. These steroids are chemically related to natural androgens with less androgen effect but with powerful effects on protein, muscle and bone build up. Nandrolone is the generic name. This medication is getting more difficult to acquire because it has been abused by many body builders. It causes new bone and muscle growth rapidly. It has side effects that may limit its use, such as worsening of the blood lipid profile, baldness, liver damage and masculinization.

It is given intramuscularly at a dose of 50mg every few weeks and at this dosage causes an increase in bone density of two percent per year for the first four years. Studies have not been carried on longer than four years.

Fluoride is supplemented at 40 to 80mg per day. It is popular in Europe but is considered experimental in the United States since there is a question regarding the quality of the new bone formed while it is being taken. The bone density increases by 5.5 percent yearly for the first few years.

Vitamin D is added to milk but injectable Vitamin D is used if there is malabsorption or poor absorption of calcium from the bowel. Side effects may be kidney failure and it is so effective at increasing calcium absorption that it should not be used with any other forms of therapy for osteoporosis as the blood levels of calcium will be excessively high. Vitamin D is given in doses of 7000-25,000 units daily in severe cases of osteoporosis when the benefits outweigh the risks.

Thiazide diuretics have a favorable effect on bone mass and limit bone fractures. Thiazides were found to be useful in patients who formed calcium-type kidney stones because the kidneys were throwing out too much calcium. The thiazide diuretics limit calcium excretion by the kidney to small amounts only. The dosage is 25mg per day of H.C.T.Z. (hydrochlorothiazide), the generic name. At higher doses, loss of potassium may be severe and result in heart arrhythmias. Low doses of 25mg per day protect and harden the bones up to 1-2 percent per year.

Without exercise or medication, calcium supplements after menopause do not stop the slow drainage of calcium from the bones. With very high doses of supplemental calcium (2000-2500mg), taken daily for four years, it was proved that there is only a 1.6 percent increase in bone density. These high levels cause constipation and are not recommended. At current recommended doses the bones lose density each year.

Estrogen can increase spinal bone density up to 6 percent per year for the first two years of use during menopause, then the increase is smaller.

Ipriflavone, a new medication should be available soon. Oral doses of 600mg result in increased bone mass within one year. Some nausea or diarrhea may occur but thus far has not been severe enough to stop the medication.

Can you afford to get older? Can you afford to have your bones melt away? The emotional costs of getting older can be painful due to separation, death of loved ones and loneliness, but add to these stresses the constant drain on your hard-earned savings to pay medical bills and nursing home bills and the cost is unacceptable. You owe it to yourself to be certain that you needn't depend on being rich enough to have osteoporosis. Have regular physical check-ups, follow your health care provider's suggestions and the ideas presented in this book. Read books recommended in the selected references and take control of your future.

Exercise is the solid cornerstone of osteoporosis prevention and treatment in this age group. Several medications can be helpful in severe cases where bones seem to break from trivial incidents such as coughing. Schedule an appointment with your health care provider and discuss your options. Make a goal of postponing the consequences of osteoporosis until you are 100 years old. Seize the day. Seize a full life.

... 11 ...

Frequently Asked Questions

Q. Why do women have more fractures than men?
A. The male hormone testosterone causes men's bones to become larger and more dense. In addition, men do not abruptly stop making hormones as women do at the menopause. Men lose about 1% per year of bone mass starting at 35 as women do, but women lose 3% per year for 10 years after menopause. By age 60 a woman has lost 45% of her bone mass while a man has lost 25%

Q. At what age do we reach our peak bone mass?
A. At about age 35 women reach peak bone mass. This doesn't mean you can't add bone mass later with exercise, calcium and new medications that are available.

Q. When should I have a bone density test?
A. When you stop having periods you should check your bone density. This is true if you had a hysterectomy and removal of the ovaries at age 35 or if you go through a natural menopause at about age 50.

Q. My dentist reports that my teeth are loose and wants me to have a bone density test. Can you explain the relationship between teeth and bones?

A. The mouth is one of the first places that osteoporosis may appear. Your dentist often is the first person to spot a change in bone health based on weaker density and loss of strength in the jaw bone. The jaw bone should hold your teeth firmly in place. Osteoporosis may first be diagnosed as pyorrhea, gum disorders, or, as it actually is called, osteoporosis of the mouth.

If you have developed osteoporosis of the mouth it means your jaw has become porous, less able to hold your teeth firmly in place. If your teeth begin to move, your gums may become inflamed and may recede, opening the path for bacteria and infection.

While tooth or gum problems aren't sure signs of osteoporosis, they do bear looking into. Periodontal disease is the major cause of tooth loss as we age, and it is more common in women than in men. Its wise to find out whether you're dealing with a dental hygiene problem or an early signal of bone loss.

Q. How soon after a hysterectomy should I start estrogen?

A. If your ovaries were removed along with your uterus, you will experience immediate hot flashes and general discomfort. This is due to the rapid withdrawal of estrogen from your system. Many surgeons give an injection of long-acting estrogen at the time of surgery to prevent hot flashes. If you are a candidate for estrogen, start it as soon as possible if you have had your ovaries removed.

Q. I had a hysterectomy one year ago but my ovaries were left in. Why do I have hot flashes?

A. Many surgeons say that during a hysterectomy, the blood supply to the ovaries may be decreased and the ovaries may stop producing normal amounts of estrogen. A blood test can be performed that measures your estrogen.

Q. Which bone density test should I have performed?

A. The test you have will depends on what resources are available in your community. DEXA X-ray tests are the most popular at this time but this may not be available in your community. Since the spine and hip are the target areas for fractures, ask your physician which tests are available that will test these areas. Dual Photon (DPA) or

Quantitative Cat Scanning (QCT) will check these areas of bone.

Q. Why do spine and hip fractures occur so commonly?
A. The vertebral bones and the top of the hip bone are made up of trabecular or spongy bone that loses its density rapidly. Other long bones of the body are made up of cortical bone that is thicker and less prone to fracture.

Q. I am taking Verapamil, a medicine called a calcium channel blocker. Will this block calcium from being absorbed?
A. Calcium channel blockers are medications taken for treatment of rapid heart rhythms, high blood pressure and migraine headaches. They block calcium flow in the tiny muscles of the small arteries but will not prevent you from absorbing calcium.

Q. I'm a long distance runner, 31 years old. My menstrual periods vanished along with most of my body fat while I was in training. Now, my doctor tells me that I have amenorrhea, my monthly period stopped. I'm in danger, my doctor says, because the slowing down of estrogen production from losing my period on top of having an athlete's body is starving my bones. Is that true?
A. Absolutely! Women who exercise greatly are at maximum risk for osteoporosis because they have experienced prolonged periods of diminished estrogen. Estrogen, remember, directly affects as many as three hundred different body processes. Among the processes, it encourages our bones to maintain their equilibrium in the bone-remodeling process — putting bone back in the same proportion as it is destroyed. Without estrogen, bone is melting away and is not being replaced. This negative balance in your bone bank must be reversed to bring back your periods, and encourage normal bone remodeling. By all means get a bone density test to find out what damage has been done so that you may reverse it. A change in your diet, adding calcium-rich foods, additional calcium, or hormone supplementation may be called for.

Q. Is it true that people with diabetes have softer bones than normal?
A. Yes, diabetes causes bone density to be about 10% lower than average so if you have diabetes and are menopausal, request a bone density test to see how dense your bones are.

Q. My insurance doesn't pay for bone density tests and my doctor says I am high risk for osteoporosis. What can I do?

A. You can contact your insurance company representative and write a letter requesting the procedure. Also ask your doctor to write a letter explaining your circumstances. If this fails, contact your congressional representative. If this fails you may have to pay for the test personally. The money spent is much less than one week in a nursing home after a hip fracture.

Q. My pharmacist said not to take my calcium with fiber rich foods like cereals or with my iron tablets? How much of the calcium is bound up by fiber and iron?

A. Calcium does bind with the fiber in cereals and with iron but the exact amount of binding is unknown. If you count the calcium milligrams in your milk on your cereal, it will likely be lower than anticipated. Separate your calcium and iron tablets by a few hours to increase absorption.

Q. Doesn't it seem crazy to make estrogen from horse urine and expect women to swallow that?

A. You're not getting undiluted horse urine in the estrogen compound that goes into Premarin, the leading estrogen replacement drug. Premarin, made by Ayerst Company, is made from pregnant mare's urine. The test of its effectiveness has been proven by the fact that it prevents osteoporosis. Premarin has been around a long time but newer hormones including estrogen patches are shown to prevent osteoporosis also. Estrace, a newer feminine hormone, replaces the same estrogen that is lost at menopause through the hormone 17-Beta-Estradiol. Discuss these hormones with your doctor to learn your treatment options.

Q. Do noisy, creaking, and often painful joints indicate bone loss? What can I do to stop the deterioration if that's what it is?

A. I am beginning to believe that creaking bones and other forms of joint pain are among the symptoms of midlife in women that we know the least about. The studies I've read show that as many as half of the women surveyed complained of either creaking or painful joints. Troubling joints with or before the first hot flashes, may be related to a reduction of cortisone, a substance, acting like oil, naturally secreted by our adrenal glands to keep joints moving freely. My best advise is for you to check out your protesting joints with your physician to make sure that you do not have an under-lying medical condition such as fibromyalgia (an arthritis-related, painful condition), arthritis, or osteoarthritis. Once he has ruled out these problems he might suggest extra Vitamin B6, Vitamin E, or Vitamin C and cod-liver oil (Vitamin D). Many women have told me that cod-liver oil works to alleviate painful and creaking joints. It certainly wouldn't hurt for you to begin a program of gentle stretching of the muscles around the joints to reduce the stress or tension on them.

Q. Can I avoid estrogen and still have hard bones?
A. Studies show that calcium supplements and exercise can restore some bone density even without estrogen. To be sure, obtain a bone density test at menopause and two years later to monitor your bone density. If your bones are staying hard over a two year period after menopause, your program is working.

Q. Is there a relationship between arthritis and osteoporosis?
A. Not that we know of. Arthritis is a joint disease and osteoporosis is a bone disease. Arthritis, which is a term used to designate many kinds of diseases, should not be con-fused with the most common form of arthritis called osteoarthritis. This is a condition that usually worsens slowly with age and can start out so deceptively that its effects are undetectable for many years. Most often it is seen as an enlargement, or thickening, of the bone of the joint. Arthritis can be seen most easily in the enlargement of the joints of the fingers. The most serious form of osteoarthritis is usually in the knee and hip joints.

Although osteoarthritis may be disabling, it is not related to osteoporosis, though people with osteoarthritic hips rarely break them. People with osteoporosis, in contrast to osteoarthritic persons, are frequently smaller in build, stooped, and their bones are porous and frail.

People suffering from osteoarthritis must still be concerned about calcium consumption and exercise, and often joint replacement surgery is performed to keep them active.

Rheumatoid arthritis is a different story. A crippling joint disease that is diag-nosed by a blood test, arthritis tends to cause more serious problems with osteoporo-sis than people in the general population. Often rheumatoid arthritis sufferers have less calcium circulating in their bloodstreams; they frequently are more sedentary because of their painful joints and often they take pain medications, such as cortisone-like drugs, which block calcium absorption. As a result, they break their hips and other bones more often.

Q. I have an underactive thyroid gland and for many years I have taken a drug called Synthroid to replace my deficiency of thyroid hormone. Does this put me at risk for osteoporosis?

There is little disagreement that thyroid hormone production can affect bone metabolism. An underactive thyroid gland, a condition called hypothyroidism, is usually treated with a drug such as Synthroid, which can literally "knock out" your own thyroid gland's production system, by replacing it. In doing so, if the levels are not right it can have the same effect on your system as if you were hyperthyroid, that is, secreting too much thyroid hormone, which is scientifically known to put you at a higher risk for osteoporosis. A simple, fairly new blood test, the Ultra Sensitive TSH (Thyroid Stimulating Hormone), can let your physician know whether the dose you're taking is right for you. If you are taking the correct amount of thyroid hormone replacement, bone loss shouldn't be a problem.

Q. If arthritis medications contribute to bone loss, what other drugs have a negative effect on bones?

A. Corticosteroids are culprits which by interfering with the balance in our bone remodeling system may increase the risk of developing osteoporosis. Used to reduce inflammation and as immunosuppressive agents, corticosteroids are widely used to treat asthma, arthritis, lupus erythematosus, osteoarthritis, and other conditions.

Aluminum-containing antacids may be harmful to your bones. When aluminum is present, extra calcium is removed from your body because the aluminum combines with the body's phosphorus and the calcium, drawing them into your urine. Loss of calcium can weaken your bones. Aluminum also deposits in bones, causing osteomalacia (a softening of bones). Other drugs that may have negative effects on our bones include those that treat certain cardiac irregularities or prevent seizures, such as phenytoin and barbiturate anticonvulsants. Also, methotrexate, a drug used in cancer and immune disorders; cyclosporine A, a medication used following organ transplantation; and gonadotropin-releasing hormones, often used to treat endometriosis are culprits. Over-the-counter preparations can harm your bones as well. Discuss your risk of osteoporosis with your doctor. He may determine if a bone-density test should be done for you. If you are at risk of losing bone and are postmenopausal, maybe estrogen replacement therapy plus extra calcium and exercise should be considered.

Glossary

<u>Biphosphonates</u> Prescription medication that hardens the bone by preventing the osteoclasts (bone crunchers) from destroying bone cells.

<u>Bone</u> <u>Mass</u> The amount of bone protein and calcium in the bone. It reaches its peak amount at about age 35.

<u>Calcium</u> The most important mineral that lines up along the bone protein lines to harden the bones.

<u>Calcitonin</u> A thyroid hormone that prevents bone breakdown. The medically useful type is from salmon and is given in shot form daily or every other day. It usually hardens the bone by 8% the first year and less thereafter.

<u>Dual</u> <u>Photon</u> <u>Absorptiometry</u> <u>(DPA)</u> An X-ray test that sends out photons from two sources to measure bone density.

Dual Energy X-ray Absorptiometry (DEXA) An X-ray test available in larger medical centers that measures bone mass with less radiation and more accuracy than other methods.

Dowager's Hump The bulging in the mid to upper back of women who have had compression fractures. It causes a stooped posture.

Estrogen The feminine hormone produced by the ovaries that slows or prevents bone loss while it is being taken.

Fluoride A chemical compound under investigation, thought to create more dense bones but not always stronger bones. It has many side effects and is not encouraged by most physicians.

Osteoblast An active bone cell that builds bone.

Osteoclast An active bone cell that destroys bone. Usually the osteoblast and osteoclast activity are in harmony. In osteoporosis, the osteoclast activity is increased.

Osteoporosis A disease of low density of bone which frequently results in fractures. Type 1 is from lack of estrogen. Type 2 is from aging and usually occurs in the late 70s and 80s.

Quantitative Computerized Tomography (QCT) An X-ray technique to measure bone density. It is an accurate technique but is associated with a high dose of radiation.

Vertebrae The bones of the spine. Usually the lower thoracic and upper lumbar vertebrae are affected by osteoporosis resulting in compression fractures and the Dowager's hump in the mid to upper back.

Vitamin D The sunlight vitamin. Exposure to 20 minutes of sunlight daily will convert the oils in the skin to this vitamin. Vitamin D improves the uptake of calcium from the intestines into the bloodstream.

Selected References

Aloia, John F., M.D., *Osteoporosis,* Leisure Press, Champaign, Illinois, 1989.

Appleton, Nancy, Ph.D., *Healthy Bones; What You Should Know About Osteoporosis,* Avery Publishers, Garden City, New York, 1991.

Bailey, Covert and Bishop. Lea, *The Fit Or Fat Woman*, Houghton Mifflin, Boston, 1989,

Decker, John, M.D., *Understanding And Managing Osteoporosis,* Avon Books, New York, 1988.

Francis. R.M., *Osteoporosis; Pathogenesis and Management,* Kluwer Academic Publishers, Boston. 1990.

Friedan. Betty, *The Fountain of Age,* Simon and Schuster, New York, 1993.

Gray, Timothy J., D.O. *Back Works; The Illustrated Guide To How Your Back Works And What To Do When It Doesn't,* BookPartners, Seattle 1993.

Greer, Germaine, *The Change; Women, Aging and the Menopause.* Fawcett Columbine, New York, 1991.

Henkel, Gretchen, *Making The Estrogen Decision.* Fawcett Columbine, New York, New York.

Jacobowitz. Ruth S., *150 Most Asked Questions About Osteoporosis,* Hearst Books, New York, 1993.

Jovanovic, Lois. M.D. with Levert. Suzanne, *A Woman Doctor's Guide To Menopause,* Hyperion Press, New York, 1993.

McIlwain, Harris H., M.D. et al. *Osteoporosis ; Prevention, Treatment, Management,* John Wiley and Sons, New York,1988.

Notelovitz, Morris, M.D,. and Ware, Marsha, *Stand Tall; Every Woman's Guide to Preventing Osteoporosis,* Triad Publishing Co., Gainesville, Florida. 1982.

O'Leary Cobb. Janine, *Understanding Menopause, Answers and Advice for Women in the Prime of Life,* Penguin Books, New York, 1993.

Rinzler. Carol Ann, *Estrogen And Breast Cancer*, MacMillan Publishing, New York, New York.

Rozek, Jan, R.N. *Keys To Understanding Osteoporosis,* Barrons, Hauppaugen, New York, 1992.

Sachs. Judith, *What You Can Do About Osteoporosis*, Dell Publishers, New York, 1993.

Sheehy. Gail, *The Silent Passage,* Pocket Books, New York, 1993.

Wolfe, Sidney M., M.D., *Women's Health Alert,* Addison-Wesley Reading, Mass., 1990.

Articles From The Medical Literature

Breast Cancer In Japanese And Caucasian Women In Hawaii. *National Cancer Institute Monograph,* 1985. Pages 191-196.

Calcium Supplementation And Bone Mineral Density In Adolescent Girls. *Journal Of The American Medical Association,* August 18, 1993. Pages 841-844.

The Effect Of Postmenopausal Estrogen Therapy On Bone Density In Elderly Women. *The New England Journal Of Medicine,* October 1993. Pages 1141-1146.

Menopausal Estrogen Replacement Therapy And Breast Cancer. *Archives of Internal Medicine,* January, 1991. Pages 67-72.

Non-contraceptive Estrogens And The Risk Of Breast Cancer in Women. *British Journal of Cancer,* 1986. Pages 853-858.

Osteoporosis: A Clinical Overview Of Diagnosis And Therapy. *The Journal Of Musculoskeletal Medicine,* August 1993. Pages 31-39.

The Roles Of Estrogen And Progesterone In Breast And Genital Cancer. *Journal Of The American Medical Association,* 1962. Pages 327-331.

Surgically Confirmed Gallbladder Disease, Venous Thromboembolism, And Breast Tumors In Relation To Post-menopausal Estrogen Therapy. Boston Collaborative Drug Surveillance Program. *New England Journal Of Medicine,* 1974. Pages 15-19.

The Waning Effect Of Postmenopausal Estrogen Therapy On Osteoporosis. *The New England Journal Of Medicine,* October 1993. Pages 1192-1193.

Abraham, G. et al. A total dietary program emphasizing magnesium instead of calcium. Effect on the mineral density of calcaneous (heel) bone in postmenopausal women on hormonal therapy. *Journal of Reproductive Medicine.* 1990; 35: 503-507.

Arnett, T. R., Dempster, D. W. Effect of pH on bone resorption by rat osteoclasts in vitro. *Endocrinology* 1986; 119:119-124.

Atik, O. S. Zinc and senile osteoporosis. *Journal American Geriatric Society.* 1983; 31: 790-791.

Barzel, U. S. Acid-induced osteoporosis: an experimental model of human osteoporosis. *Calcified Tissue Research* 1976; 21:Suppl: 417-22.

Boyce, W. J., Vessey, M. P. Rising incidence of fracture of the proximal femur. *Lancet.* 1985; 1:150-151.

Bushinsky D. A., Sessler N. E. Critical role of bicarbonate in calcium release from bone. *American Journal of Physiology* 1992; 263:F510-515.

Charles, P., Poser, J. W., et al. Estimation of bone turnover evaluated by 47Ca-kinetics; efficiency of serum bone gamma-carboxyglutamic acid-containing protein, serum alkaline phosphatase, and urinary hydroxyproline excretion. *Journal Clinical Investigation.* 1985; 76:2254-58.

Christiansen, C., Riis, B.J.: 17 Beta-estradiol And Continuous Norethisterone: A Unique Treatment For Established Osteoporosis In Elderly Women. *Journal of Clinical Endocrinology Metabolism* 71:836-841, 1989.

Cohen, L. and Kitzes, R. Infrared spectroscopy and magnesium content of bone mineral in osteoporotic women. *Israel: Journal of Medical Science.* 1981; 17: 1123-1125.

Deacon A. C., Hulme P., et al. Estimation of whole body bone resorption rate: a comparison of urinary total hydroxyproline excretion with two radioisotopic tracer methods in osteoporosis. *Clinical Chimica Acta.* 1987; 166:297-306.

Epstein S. Serum and urinary markers of bone remodeling: assessment of bone turnover. *Endocrin Review* 1988; 9:437-49.

Frithiof, L. et al. The relationship between marginal bone loss and serum zinc levels. *Acta Medica Scandinavia.* 1980; 207: 67-70.

Knapen, M., et al. The effect of Vitamin K supplementation on circulating osteocalcin (bone GLA protein) and urinary calcium excretion. *Annals of Internal Medicine.* 1989; 111:1001-1005.

Krieger, N.S., et al. Acidosis inhibits osteoblastic and stimulates osteoclastic activity in vitro. *American Journal of Physiology* 1992; 262:F442-F448.

Lees, B., et al. Differences in proximal femur bone density of two centuries. *Lancet.* 1993; 341:673-675.

Lindsay, R., Tohme, J.F: Estrogen Treatment Of Patients With Established Postmenopausal Osteoporosis. *Obstetrics and Gynecology* 76:290-295, 1990.

Lukert, B.P., Johnson, B.E., Robinson, R.G.: Estrogen And Progesterone Replacement Therapy Reduces Glucocorticoid Induced Bone Loss. *Journal of Bone and Mineral Research.* 7:1063-1069, 1992.

Lutz, J. Calcium balance and acid-base status of women as affected by increased protein intake and by sodium bicarbonate ingestion. *American Journal Clinical Nutrition* 1984; 39:281-88.

Marsh, A. G., et al. Cortical bone density of adult lacto-ovo-vegetarian and omnivorous women. *Journal American Diet Association.* 1980; 76:148-151.

Mena, I. The role of manganese in human disease. *Annals of Clinical Laboratory Science* 1974; 4:487-491.

Menchen, H.L. Exeunt Omnes. *Smart Set* 1919; 60:138-45.

Mulder, H, Snelder, H.A.A.: Effect Of Cyclical Etidronate Regimen On Prophylaxis Of Bone Loss Of Glucocorticoid (Prednisone) Therapy In Postmenopausal Women. *Journal of Bone and Mineral Research.* 7(Suppl 1): S331, 1992.

Need, A.G., Horowitz, M, Bridges, A., et al: Effects Of Nandrolone Decanoate And Antiresorptive Therapy On Vertebral Density In Osteoporotic Postmenopausal Women. *Archives of Internal Medicine* 149: 57-60, 1989.

Raloff, J. Reasons for boning up on manganese. *Science News.* 1986; 130 (27 Sept.): 199.

Rosenstock, H., et al. Chronic manganism. Neurologic and laboratory studies during treatment with levodopa. *Journal American Medical Association.* 1973; 217: 1354-1358.

Schroeder, J. A. Losses of vitamins and trace minerals resulting from processing and preservation of foods. *American Journal of Clinical Nutrition.* 1971; 24:562-573.

Saffar, J. L., et al. Osteoporotic effect of a high carbohydrate diet in golden hamsters. *Archives of Oral Biology.* 1981; 26: 393-397.

Storm, T., Thamsborg, G., Steiniche, T., et al: Effect Of Intermittent Cyclical Etidronate Therapy On Bone Mass And Fracture Rate In Women With Postmenopausal Osteoporosis. *New England Journal Of Medicine* 322: 1265-1271, 1990.

Yudkin, J., *Sweet and Dangerous.* Bantam Books, New York, 1973.